Blunt Trauma Injuries in the Athlete

Editor

THOMAS M. DEBERARDINO

CLINICS IN
SPORTS MEDICINE

www.sportsmed.theclinics.com

Consulting Editor
MARK D. MILLER

April 2013 • Volume 32 • Number 2

ELSEVIER

1600 John F. Kennedy Boulevard • Suite 1800 • Philadelphia, Pennsylvania, 19103

http://www.theclinics.com

CLINICS IN SPORTS MEDICINE Volume 32, Number 2
April 2013 ISSN 0278-5919, ISBN-13: 978-1-4557-7332-9

Editor: Jennifer Flynn-Briggs

Clinics in Sports Medicine (ISSN 0278-5919) is published quarterly by Elsevier Inc., 360 Park Avenue South, New York, NY 10010-1710. Months of issue are January, April, July, and October. Business and Editorial Offices: 1600 John F. Kennedy Blvd., Ste. 1800, Philadelphia, PA 19103-2899. Customer Service Office: 3251 Riverport Lane, Maryland Heights, MO 63043. Periodicals postage paid at New York, NY and additional mailing offices. Subscription prices are $324.00 per year (US individuals), $523.00 per year (US institutions), $159.00 per year (US students), $367.00 per year (Canadian individuals), $631.00 per year (Canadian institutions), $222.00 (Canadian students), $446.00 per year (foreign individuals), $631.00 per year (foreign institutions), and $222.00 per year (foreign students). Foreign air speed delivery is included in all *Clinics* subscription prices. All prices are subject to change without notice. **POSTMASTER:** Send address changes to *Clinics in Sports Medicine*, Elsevier Health Sciences Division, Subscription Customer Service, 3251 Riverport Lane, Maryland Heights, MO 63043. Customer Service (orders, claims, online, change of address): Elsevier Health Sciences Division, Subscription Customer Service, 3251 Riverport Lane, Maryland Heights, MO 63043. Tel: 1-800-654-2452 (U.S. and Canada); 314-447-8871 (outside U.S. and Canada). Fax: 314-447-8029. E-mail: journalscustomerservice-usa@elsevier.com (for print support); journalsonlinesupport-usa@elsevier.com (for online support).

Reprints. For copies of 100 or more of articles in this publication, please contact the Commercial Reprints Department, Elsevier Inc., 360 Park Avenue South, New York, NY 10010-1710. Tel.: 212-633-3812; Fax: 212-462-1935; E-mail: reprints@elsevier.com.

Clinics in Sports Medicine is covered in *MEDLINE/PubMed (Index Medicus) Current Contents/Clinical Medicine, Excerpta Medica,* and *ISI/Biomed.*

Printed and bound by CPI Group (UK) Ltd, Croydon, CR0 4YY

Transferred to digital print 2012

Contributors

CONSULTING EDITOR

MARK D. MILLER, MD
S. Ward Casscells Professor of Orthopaedic Surgery, University of Virginia; Team Physician, JBJS Deputy Editor for Sports Medicine, Director, Miller Review Course, James Madison University, Charlottesville, Virginia

EDITOR

THOMAS M. DEBERARDINO, MD
Associate Professor, Department of Orthopaedic Surgery, New England Musculoskeletal Institute, University of Connecticut Health Center; Team Physician, Orthopaedic Consultant, Athletic Department, University of Connecticut, Farmington, Connecticut

AUTHORS

GISELLE A. AERNI, MD
Associate Fellowship Director, Primary Care Sports Medicine, University of Connecticut, Hartford, Connecticut; Assistant Professor, Family Medicine, University of Connecticut Health Center, Farmington, Connecticut; Team Physician, University of Connecticut, Storrs, Connecticut; Team Physician, WNBA CT Sun, Uncasville, Connecticut

JEFFREY ANDERSON, MD, FACSM
Director of Sports Medicine and Head Team Physician, Medical Director for Research Human Performance Laboratory, Division of Athletics, University of Connecticut, Storrs, Connecticut

DEENA C. CASIERO, MD
Attending Primary Care Sports Medicine Department, ProHEALTH Care Associates, Lake Success, New York; Medical Consultant and Associate Team Physician, USA Seven's Women's Rugby, Colorado; Team Physician, Hofstra University, Hempstead, New York; Tournament Physician, US Open Tennis Championships, Flushing, New York; Associate Team Physician, New York Islanders, Hempstead Turnpike, Uniondale, New York

THOMAS M. DEBERARDINO, MD
Associate Professor, Department of Orthopaedic Surgery, New England Musculoskeletal Institute, University of Connecticut Health Center; Team Physician, Orthopaedic Consultant, Athletic Department, University of Connecticut, Farmington, Connecticut

KYLEF EAGLES, DO
University of Massachusetts Sports Medicine, Amherst, Massachusetts

JEFFREY P. FEDEN, MD
Assistant Professor, Department of Emergency Medicine, Alpert Medical School of Brown University, Providence, Rhode Island

LAURA FRALICH, MD
University of Massachusetts Sports Medicine, Amherst, Massachusetts

IVETTE GUTTMANN, MD
Primary Care Sports Medicine Fellowship, Division of Internal Medicine and Pediatrics, Department of Medicine, Albany Medical College, Albany, New York

MATTHEW HALL, DO
Primary Care Sports Medicine Fellow, Department of Family Medicine, University of Connecticut, Hartford, Connecticut

STANLEY R. HUNTER, MD
Resident, Department of Family Medicine, University of Vermont College of Medicine, Burlington, Vermont

JESSICA M. INTRAVIA, BS, MHA
MD Candidate Class of 2013, School of Medicine, University of Connecticut, Farmington, Connecticut

HAMISH A. KERR, MD, MSc, FAAP
Primary Care Sports Medicine Fellowship Director, Associate Professor Medicine, Division Internal Medicine/Pediatrics, Department of Medicine, Albany Medical College, Latham, New York

TIMOTHY S. LISHNAK, MD, CAQSM
Assistant Professor, Department of Family Medicine, University of Vermont College of Medicine, Burlington, Vermont

DAVID K. LISLE, MD, CAQSM
Assistant Professor, Division of Sports Medicine, Department of Orthopaedics and Rehabilitation; Department of Family Medicine, University of Vermont College of Medicine, Burlington, Vermont

MELISSA MASCARO, MD
Sports Medicine Fellow, Department of Sport Medicine, St Francis Hospital, University of Connecticut, Hartford, Connecticut

ANDRIA M. POWERS, MD
Resident, Department of Radiology, University of Vermont College of Medicine, Burlington, Vermont

J. HERBERT STEVENSON, MD, CAQ Sports Medicine
Chief, Division of Sports Medicine; Director, Sports Medicine Fellowship, University of Massachusetts Medical School, Department of Family Medicine and Community Health, University of Massachusetts Sports Medicine, Amherst, Massachusetts

THOMAS H. TROJIAN, MD
Director of Injury Prevention and Sports Outreach, Orthopaedics, UCHC/NEMSI; Director of Sports Medicine Fellowship Program, Family Medicine, UCHC, Farmington; Team Physician, Department of Athletics, University of Connecticut, Storrs, Connecticut

TRACEY A. VIOLA, DO
Family Practice and Sports Medicine, Lake Placid Health Center, Lake Placid, New York

Contents

Bladder injury should be suspected when trauma is followed by gross hematuria, suprapubic or abdominal pain, and difficulty in voiding or the inability to void. Bladder rupture with blunt abdominal trauma is uncommon; however, because of its high mortality rate, recognition of the early signs and symptoms can be life saving. The most common type of injury is a bladder contusion, which is a diagnosis of exclusion. Extraperitoneal bladder ruptures are almost exclusively associated with a pelvic fracture.

Male genital trauma is a rare but potentially serious sports injury. Although such an injury can occur by many different mechanisms, including falls, collisions, straddle injuries, kicks, and equipment malfunction, the clinical presentation is typically homogeneous, characterized by pain and swelling. Almost all sports-related male genital injury comes from blunt force trauma, with involvement of scrotal structures far more common than penile structures. Most injuries can be treated conservatively, but catastrophic testicular injury must first be ruled out. Despite being relatively uncommon compared with other sports injuries, more than half of all testicular injuries are sustained during sports.

Pulmonary injuries from blunt thoracic trauma are seen regularly with high-energy mechanisms but described less frequently in association with sports. Pneumothorax, hemothorax, pneumomediastinum, and pulmonary contusion are uncommon with athletic participation and often follow a benign clinical course. Life-threatening complications may arise, and athletes with chest trauma deserve close attention. Appropriate diagnosis is suggested by history and physical examination; conventional chest radiography is preferred as the initial imaging study but has limitations. Use of CT for trauma has improved diagnostic sensitivity for occult injury, although this may not alter management or outcomes. Return to play is guided by resolution of symptoms and radiographic findings.

This article is meant to provide physicians with a working definition of blunt cardiac contusions as well as mechanism of injury for blunt cardiac contusions and the differential diagnoses. It is also meant to help physicians with management and plan of care. After a thorough history and physical examination, the implementation of prompt CPR and prehospital automatic external defibrillator use has been shown to increase the survival rate.

Closed head injuries vary from the very minor to the catastrophic. It is often difficult to differentiate the severity at initial presentation. Serial assessment is very valuable. Awareness of facial injuries is aided by familiarity with facial bone anatomy and the clinical presentation of orbital, zygomatic, maxillary, and mandibular fracture. Functional injury such as concussion may coexist with other injuries. This article will discuss closed head trauma and outline specific injuries to the face, brain, skull, and its surroundings.

Eye injuries in sports have an estimated incidence near 15%. These injuries can have a wide range of severity with a risk profile that is different for each individual sport. It is important to screen for and protect any functionally one-eyed athletes before athletic participation. Protective eyewear has been proposed in many sports, but outcomes data on its effectiveness are limited. Several blunt visual trauma injuries and their management are reviewed, and tools to have in the sideline bag and a few different ophthalmologic medicines are discussed.

Understanding basic ear anatomy and function allows an examiner to quickly and accurately identify at-risk structures in patients with head and ear trauma. External ear trauma (ie, hematoma or laceration) should be promptly treated with appropriate injury-specific techniques. Tympanic membrane injuries have multiple mechanisms and can often be conservatively treated. Temporal bone fractures are a common cause of ear trauma and can be life threatening. Facial nerve injuries and hearing loss can occur in ear trauma.

Thigh contusions are common injuries in sports, and the thigh is a very common location for sports-related muscle contusions. Treatment starts with placement of the knee in 120 of flexion for 24 hours. Nonsteroidal anti-inflammatory drugs can be detrimental to the healing if used for more than 48 to 72 hours, and glucocorticosteroids should be avoided. Early treatment with knee flexion to 120 degrees is very important, and is followed by range-of-motion exercises and advancement of activity. Early proper treatment is the key to success. Complications of myositis ossificans and compartment syndrome need to be considered.

The term, *hip pointer*, is applied in the setting of a blunt trauma injury to the iliac crest. It typically occurs in contact and collision sports and can cause significant pain and loss of practice or game time. A direct blow results in subperiosteal edema with hematoma formation within surrounding muscle or soft tissue and bone contusion of the iliac crest. Conservative management with compression, ice, antiinflammatories, and rehabilitation exercises are successful in treating hip pointers. Injection therapy with the use of local anesthetic can be helpful in minimizing pain and increasing function to allow more rapid return to play.

CLINICS IN SPORTS MEDICINE

FORTHCOMING ISSUES

July 2013
MRI in Sports Medicine
Timothy G. Sanders, MD, *Editor*

October 2013
Unicompartmental Knee Arthroplasty
Kevin Plancher, MD, and
Albert Dunn, DO, *Editors*

RECENT ISSUES

January 2013
Anatomic ACL Reconstruction
Freddie H. Fu, MD, DSc(Hon), and
Volker Musahl, MD, *Editors*

October 2012
Rotator Cuff Surgery
Stephen F. Brockmeier, MD, *Editor*

July 2012
Spinal Injuries in the Athlete
Pierre A. d'Hemecourt, MD, and
Lyle J. Micheli, MD, *Editors*

Foreword

Blunt Trauma Injuries in the Athlete

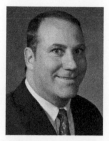

Mark D. Miller, MD
Consulting Editor

Let's be blunt about it … there really isn't a lot of information out there on how to deal with blunt trauma. This is a growing concern because the speed and intensity of play in a variety of sports, and the associated injuries, have continued to escalate. Therefore, I invited Dr Thomas DeBerardino, who has extensive experience on this topic from his career in the military to include a stent as the Chief of Sports Medicine at West Point, to organize an issue of *Clinics in Sports Medicine* on this topic. As usual, Tommy came through with flying colors!

This treatise on blunt injuries includes the whole gambit of blunt trauma including abdominal, solid organ, cardiopulmonary, head, musculoskeletal, and yes, even the dreaded GU injuries. It is well done and well organized and is a mandatory book to have handy in your training room. My thanks to Dr DeBerardino and his crew for an outstanding effort!

Mark D. Miller, MD
S. Ward Casscells Professor of Orthopaedic Surgery
University of Virginia
Team Physician, James Madison University
400 Ray C. Hunt Drive, Suite 330
Charlottesville, VA 22908-0159, USA

E-mail address:
MDM3P@hscmail.mcc.virginia.edu

Clin Sports Med 32 (2013) xi
http://dx.doi.org/10.1016/j.csm.2013.01.001
0278-5919/13/$ – see front matter © 2013 Published by Elsevier Inc.

Preface

Blunt Trauma Injuries

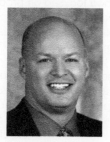

Thomas M. DeBerardino, MD
Editor

The evaluation and management of sports-related blunt trauma injuries is an important area that interfaces the sports medicine world with many other subspecialty areas of medicine. The goal of this special focus issue is to help keep physicians that care for athletes up to date regarding the latest developments pertaining to new technology to hasten diagnosis and preferred management of blunt trauma injuries.

The authors of this issue are all directly involved with treating athletes on the sidelines, the clinic, or the operating room. Another notable common thread among the authors is that they all have been or still are alumni or faculty of either our primary care sports medicine fellowship or orthopaedic sports medicine fellowship at the University of Connecticut Health Center.

All articles encompass a succinct review of the recent literature and add information regarding the use of newer technologies, such as advanced ultrasound imaging, where appropriate. Topics covered include blunt trauma of the lung, heart, abdomen, liver, spleen, genitourinary system, hip and thigh, and even the eye and ear. In addition, a timely update dealing with closed head injuries is also included.

Thomas M. DeBerardino, MD
University of Connecticut Health Center
Department of Orthopaedic Surgery
New England Musculoskeletal Institute
University of Connecticut Athletic Department
263 Farmington Avenue, MARB4
Farmington, CT 06034, USA

E-mail address:
tdeber@uchc.edu

Clin Sports Med 32 (2013) xiii
http://dx.doi.org/10.1016/j.csm.2013.01.002
0278-5919/13/$ – see front matter © 2013 Published by Elsevier Inc.

Evaluation of Blunt Abdominal Trauma

Jessica M. Intravia, BS, MHA[a],*, Thomas M. DeBerardino, MD[b]

KEYWORDS

- Blunt abdominal trauma • Sports medicine • Athlete

KEY POINTS

- The sports medicine physician needs to be able to triage athletes with blunt abdominal trauma and to recommend proper postinjury care.
- The mechanism of injury and corresponding examination findings may aid the physician in assessing the extent of the athlete's injury.
- Benign injuries include diaphragmatic spasms and rectus abdominis hematomas.
- Potentially serious injuries may involve the liver, spleen, kidneys, or pancreas.

INTRODUCTION

In 1981, Bergqvist and colleagues[1] estimated that 10% of all abdominal injuries resulted from sport-related trauma. Since then, athletic pursuits have continued to become a popular American pastime. From 1988 to 2004, female participation in National Collegiate Athletic Association (NCAA) championship sports has increased 80% and male participation has increased 20%.[2] **Table 1** reports the percentage of abdominal wall injuries from the 2004–2005 NCAA's injury surveillance system.[3]

The sports medicine physician needs to be familiar with the signs and symptoms of abdominal injury when evaluating players on the sideline. These types of injuries tend to be more common in contact or collision sports, such as hockey, football, and soccer, but have also been reported in noncontact sports, such as cycling, skiing, snowboarding, and surfing. Indirect sport-related trauma has also been reported in baseball and lacrosse from a ball striking the abdomen.[4]

First, the sideline physician should differentiate benign from potentially life-threatening abdominal injuries and determine the disposition of the player. Should the injured player return to play, be removed from competition, or be transported for further evaluation?

[a] School of Medicine, University of Connecticut School of Medicine, 263 Farmington Avenue, MARB4, Farmington, CT 06034-4037, USA; [b] Department of Orthopaedic Surgery, University of Connecticut Health Center, 263 Farmington Avenue, MARB4, Farmington, CT 06034-4037, USA
* Corresponding author.
E-mail address: jintravia@gmail.com

Clin Sports Med 32 (2013) 211–218
http://dx.doi.org/10.1016/j.csm.2012.12.001
0278-5919/13/$ – see front matter © 2013 Elsevier Inc. All rights reserved.

Table 1
Percentage of abdominal wall injuries from the 2004–2005 NCAA's injury surveillance system

Sport	Percentage of All Injuries	Injuries per 1000 Player Hours
Football (game/practice)	0.4/0.2	0.16/0.01
Men's basketball (game/practice)	-/0.4	-/0.02
Men's lacrosse (game/practice)	-/1.5	-/0.06
Men's soccer (game/practice)	0.4/0.2	0.09/0.01
Women's soccer (game/practice)	0.2/0.6	0.04/0.04
Men's wrestling (game/practice)	2.9/-	0.71/-
Women's volleyball (game/practice)	5.7/3.7	0.28/0.2

Data from Johnson R. Abdominal wall injuries: rectus abdominis strains, oblique strains, rectus sheath hematoma. Curr Sports Med Rep 2006;5:99–103.

One consideration is the mechanism of injury. Direct trauma often results from a blow to the abdomen. This mechanism will result in local injury and damage to the overlying skin and subcutaneous blood vessels. The depth of the injury is related to the force of the blow. In contrast, an acceleration/deceleration-type injury occurs when a moving athlete is abruptly brought to a stop, i.e. when a skier hits a barricade. This type of injury may cause complete disruption of deep organs and very few superficial signs.

Second, patients should be assessed for any signs of shock which may indicate a need for immediate intervention. Signs of shock include tachycardia, hypotension, dyspnea, diaphoresis, anxiety, and confusion. If these signs are present, transport should be arranged to the nearest medical facility. Pending the arrival of transportation, patients should remain lying supine in a modified Trendelenburg position.

Finally, the type of abdominal pain can lead to insights concerning the underlying condition and severity of injury. Considerations include immediate versus worsening pain, local versus diffuse pain, and stationary versus radiating pain. Other characteristics include the presence or absence of guarding, rigidity, rebound tenderness, and peritoneal signs. Certain physical examination findings may signal characteristic pathologic conditions. A Kehr sign demonstrates pain radiating to the left shoulder which suggests diaphragmatic irritation secondary to free fluid. The Cullen sign demonstrates a bluish periumbilical discoloration suggestive of hemoperitoneum. A Grey Turner sign demonstrates a similar bluish discoloration of the flank also suggestive of hemoperitoneum.[4]

TYPES OF INJURIES
Diaphragmatic Spasm

Oftentimes, a player will complain of "getting the wind knocked out" after a blow to the abdomen in the region of the epigastrium. This injury is the most common injury in contact and collision sports and results in dyspnea secondary to temporary diaphragmatic muscle spasm. Until the spasm resolves, the athlete may complain of difficulty breathing, which can be relieved by hip flexion and loosening of restrictive equipment or clothing. The athlete can safely return to play once breathing has normalized. However, if breathing does not normalize, concern for more serious injury should be raised.[4]

Abdominal Wall Muscle Injury

Another common abdominal injury in athletics is a contusion of the abdominal wall musculature. This injury can result from either a direct or indirect mechanism. A direct blow, such as from a helmet or shoulder pad, may result in a contusion and hematoma. An indirect mechanism, such as a sudden violent contraction of the abdominal musculature, may cause an injury of the muscle tissue. Patients will often present with pain on trunk flexion and rotation or local tenderness. The injury is usually self-limited and may be treated with rest, ice, and analgesics. If a more significant abdominal wall contusion exists, physical therapy and rehabilitation may help regain motion, strength, and endurance.[4]

Rectus Abdominis Hematoma

One type of abdominal wall contusion is a rectus abdominis hematoma. The rectus abdominis is a vertical muscle that extends the length of the abdomen from the inferior costal margin to the symphysis pubis. It functions in flexing the vertebral column and compressing the abdominal and pelvic cavities. This function assists in respiration by pulling the chest downward and depressing the lower ribs. An injury to the epigastric or large intramuscular vessels can cause hemorrhage and formation of a large hematoma between the rectus sheath.

The clinical presentation of a rectus abdominis hematoma can mimic an acute abdomen. Patients can present with sudden abdominal pain, rapid swelling, occasional nausea and vomiting, and rebound or guarding. Patients may report relief with the abdomen in a supported flexed position and worsening of the pain with active flexion. On physical examination, a tender palpable mass can often be felt below the umbilicus. Cullen sign, a bluish periumbilical discoloration suggesting hemoperitoneum, is usually seen 72 hours after injury.[3,4]

A cross table lateral radiograph may show a soft tissue mass consistent with hematoma, which can be confirmed with computed tomography (CT) of the abdomen and pelvis. Often symptoms will resolve with ice, relative rest, and analgesics. Patients should be instructed to avoid flexion of the trunk and stretching of the abdominal musculature. Large hematomas may require surgical evacuation and ligation of the epigastric artery. Athletes may return to play as symptoms allow.[5,6]

Liver Injury

The liver is the most frequently injured abdominal organ.[4] Injury can result from a direct blow and can result in a subcapsular or intraparenchymal hematoma. Deceleration injuries can result in laceration of the liver's relatively thin capsule and underlying attached parenchyma. Patients will complain of right upper quadrant pain that may radiate to the shoulder or neck. The overlying ribs may be tender and occasional guarding is seen.

Treatment depends on the extent of liver injury. The hepatic injury scale is detailed in **Table 2**. If patients are conscious and hemodynamically unstable with peritoneal signs, an emergent laparotomy should be performed. Likewise, if patients are unconscious or there are equivocal physical signs, a diagnostic peritoneal lavage (DPL) should be performed; if it is positive, a diagnostic laparotomy should follow. If patients are hemodynamically stable, radiologic evaluation with a CT scan is necessary to determine the extent of injury.

Nonoperative management includes observation with bed rest, serial abdominal examinations, and serial hemoglobin and hematocrit for 48 hours following injury. Most hemorrhages occur in the first 24 hours and delayed bleeding is rare.[7] In fact, 50% to 80% of liver injuries will stop bleeding spontaneously.[4]

In the setting of blunt abdominal trauma, correlation has been found between aspartate aminotransferase (AST) and alanine aminotransferase (ALT) levels and the severity of liver injury. In the pediatric population, Karam and colleagues[8] found that half of the

Table 2 Hepatic injury scale		
Grade	Injury	Description
I	Hematoma	Subcapsular, <10% surface area
	Laceration	Capsular tear, <1 cm parenchymal depth
II	Hematoma	Subcapsular, 10%–50% surface area
	Laceration	Laceration, 1–3 cm parenchymal depth, <10 cm length
III	Hematoma	Subcapsular, >50% surface area or expanding
		Ruptured subcapsular or parenchymal hemorrhage
		Intraparenchymal hematoma more than 10 cm or expanding
	Laceration	>3 cm Parenchymal depth
IV	Laceration	Parenchymal disruption involving 25%–75% of hepatic lobe or 1–3 Couinaud segments within a single lobe
V	Laceration	Parenchymal disruption involving >75% of hepatic lobe or >3 Couinaud segments within a single lobe
	Vascular	Juxtahepatic venous injuries
VI	Vascular	Hepatic avulsion

Data from Parks RW, Chrysos E, Diamond T. Management of liver trauma. Br J Surg 1999;86:1121–35.

children with blunt abdominal trauma have elevated AST/ALT levels even if no discernible liver injury was found on CT. In fact, Karam and colleagues[8] could not determine AST/ALT cutoff values under which liver injury could be excluded. Puranik and colleagues[9] found that in a study of adult patients with blunt abdominal trauma, an AST greater than 400 and/or an ALT greater than 250 IU/L conveyed a sensitivity and specificity for predicting liver injury of 92.9% and 100%, respectively.

Return to play is dependent on the extent of the liver injury. A simple liver laceration and subcapsular hematoma can heal in 2 to 4 months. A large, complex laceration can require up to 6 months to heal. No CT or ultrasound (US) documentation of resolved injury is necessary before returning to play unless symptoms have not fully resolved.[7]

Splenic Injury

The spleen is the most frequently injured organ in sports and the most common cause of death caused by abdominal trauma in athletes.[4] Injuries can occur in any number of ways; even trivial mechanisms can result in splenic damage. Therefore, it is crucial to keep splenic injury on the differential diagnosis of any abdominal trauma.[10] Splenic injury is 6 times more common in snowboarding accidents when compared with skiing accidents.[11] Injuries often occur as a result of direct trauma to left lower chest wall or left upper quadrant of abdomen. Infection, pregnancy, or portal hypertension results in an enlarged spleen, which is more easily injured. In children, the rib cage does not completely cover the spleen. In addition, the thoracic cage is more compliant and transmits more energy from trauma. Thus, injuries can occur with less force than would be expected in an adult. Delayed splenic rupture is less common in children because they have thick splenic capsules, elastic parenchyma, and a higher proportion of smooth muscle.[10]

Delayed rupture is more common in spleen than in liver. The incidence ranges from 1% to 8% in adults and 0% to 7.5% in children.[4] Delayed rupture is likely to result from the development of a pseudoaneurysm, splenic abscess, or from secondary tearing of the parenchyma after an adherent omentum.[4] An initial normal CT scan does not exclude the potential for delayed splenic rupture (>48 hours after injury). Although there is no clear evidence concerning the frequency of follow-up CT scans, some research suggests that follow-up scans should be obtained within the first week and then monthly until complete resolution of the injury.[12] If patients complain of worsening discomfort, a contrast CT should be considered.

Signs of splenic injury are often delayed because the splenic capsule can contain initial bleeding. Consequently, the physical examination is unreliable. The pain is initially sharp followed by a dull left-sided ache. Generalized abdominal tenderness and distension along with occasional rebound and guarding may also be present. In addition, patients may complain of pain radiating to the left or right shoulder secondary to diaphragmatic irritation from free intraperitoneal blood. Tenderness may be present over the left 10th, 11th, and 12th ribs. If splenic injury is suspected, immediate transport should be arranged because hemodynamic status can quickly change.

Further workup should include a complete blood count. An elevated leukocyte count may be present if a subcapsular hematoma develops. Imaging studies should also be obtained. A DPL can be diagnostic in a hemodynamically unstable person. Plain radiographs may show fading of the splenic outline and growing of the splenic shadow. CT scan is the current standard of care in diagnostic imaging.[4] With contrast enhancement, a splenic laceration will appear as an irregular, linear hypodensity, whereas an intrasplenic hematoma will appear as a hypodense area in a nonperfusing region of the spleen.[12]

Splenic injury can be assessed using the American Association for the Surgery of Trauma's splenic injury scale (**Table 3**). Nonoperative management of hemodynamically stable patients is preferred. If patients are hemodynamically unstable or DPL is positive, an exploratory laparotomy should be performed. Generally splenic preservation is preferred over splenectomy because splenectomy is associated with overwhelming postsplenectomy infection. Postsplenectomy patients should be vaccinated against Haemophilus influenza type B, Neisseria meningitides, and pneumococcus to prevent infection.

Controversy exists over the length of activity restriction after nonoperative management of blunt splenic injury. Generally a 3-month period of activity restriction is

Table 3
American Association for the Surgery of Trauma's splenic injury scale

Grade	Injury	Description
I	Hematoma	Subcapsular, nonexpanding, <10% surface area
	Laceration	Capsular tear, nonbleeding, <1 cm parenchymal depth
II	Hematoma	Subcapsular, nonexpanding, 10%–50% surface area
		Intraparenchymal, nonexpanding, <2 cm in diameter
	Laceration	Capsular tear, active bleeding, 1–3 cm parenchymal depth that does not involve a trabecular vessel
III	Hematoma	Subcapsular, >50% surface area or expanding
		Ruptured subcapsular hematoma with active bleeding
		Intraparenchymal hematoma >2 cm or expanding
	Laceration	>3 cm Parenchymal depth or involving trabecular vessels
IV	Hematoma	Ruptured intraparenchymal hematoma with active bleeding
	Laceration	Laceration involving segmental or hilar vessels producing major devascularization (>25% of spleen)
V	Laceration	Completely shattered spleen
	Vascular	Hilar vascular injury that devascularizes spleen

Data from Moore EE, Shackford SR, Pachter HL, et al. Organ injury scaling: spleen, liver and kidney. J Trauma 1989;29:1664–6.

recommended because most injured spleens heal within 2.0 to 2.5 months. Imaging plays no role in the return-to-play assessment because radiographic healing lags behind clinical healing. The first 3 weeks after hospital discharge should be spent mainly participating in quiet activity at home. Postsplenectomy patients may return to full activity depending on surgical incision closure and patient desire.[4]

Renal Injury

Two important indicators of severity after a suspected renal injury are hematuria and hypotension. One study of 2254 adult patients with blunt renal trauma found that no significant renal injuries were missed without gross hematuria, hypotension, or significant mechanism of injury.[13] However, hematuria alone is missing with 2% to 4% of patients with renal injuries.[14] Children are more likely than adults to sustain renal injury from blunt abdominal trauma. Proposed reasoning for this discrepancy includes greater relative size of the kidney, decreased perirenal fat, weaker abdominal musculature, and increased ribcage flexibility.[12,15]

Laboratory evaluation should include a urinary analysis, complete blood count, glucose, amylase, lipase, and human chorionic gonadotropin level. If the urinalysis shows more than 50 red blood cells per high-power field, hypotension, or significant injury mechanism, a CT pelvis should be obtained.[15] If obtained, a plain radiograph may show a lack of psoas sign on the involved side.[13] However, CT is the gold standard to evaluate for renal injury. A medial hematoma, medial extravasation of contrast on the delayed films, or lack of parenchymal contrast in the early phase suggests major renal injury. Some authors suggest that a follow-up CT scan before discharge and another in 6 to 10 weeks after injury should be performed in patients with renal injury.[12]

Return to play should not be allowed until hematuria has completely resolved. Minor renal injuries can take 2 to 6 weeks to resolve. Pediatric athletes may take longer to return. Major renal injuries can take 6 to 12 months before a player can safely return.

Pancreatic Injury

Pancreatic injury is rare in sports-related abdominal trauma, but pancreatic laceration and duct injury should be included in the differential diagnosis because it can be a cause of significant morbidity. Usually, injuries are a result of direct contact. Patients may complain of abdominal pain and tenderness that typically diminishes within the first 2 hours after injury and increases again over the intervening 6 to 8 hours. Postinjury complications often include pseudocyst formation.[16]

Management depends on the extent of pancreatic injury. Evaluation should be based on serial clinical examinations, pancreatic enzyme levels, imaging, and magnetic resonance cholangiopancreatography (MRCP) or endoscopic retrograde cholangiopancreatography (ERCP). Serum amylase levels can be elevated in any number of abdominal injuries and are neither specific nor sensitive to pancreatic injury. Serial elevation of serum amylase levels and lipase levels are more specific to pancreatic injury.[16] Imaging modalities include DPL, CT, or focused assessment with sonography for trauma (FAST) abdominal ultrasound.

There are no clear written guidelines that concern the athlete's return to play after pancreatic injury. It depends on the resolution of the disease process and symptoms.

IMAGING MODALITIES AFTER BLUNT ABDOMINAL TRAUMA

Plain radiographs are a useful starting point for most traumatic abdominal injuries. Supine and right lateral decubitus or upright chest radiographs should be performed if visceral perforation is suspected. If free air is found, operative care is necessary.

Ultrasound along with direct peritoneal lavage is a mainstay in the diagnosis of abdominal trauma. FAST is a first-line study for unstable patients and can assess free peritoneal fluid.[17] FAST has a lower effectiveness in children and fails to detect a significant number of abdominal injuries without intraperitoneal fluid.[18] Recently, CT scans have replaced US in the diagnosis of stable patients. Ultrasound imaging has been reported to have 85% sensitivity and a large operator dependent error. However, US serves as good diagnostic tool for abdominal wall injuries, such as rectus sheath hematomas.[12]

CT scan is the gold standard in evaluating abdominal trauma and the test of choice for identifying spleen, liver, and kidney injuries.[12] It is not indicated for unstable patients. Contrast-enhanced CT gives increased details, including the ability to detect subtle lacerations of the liver and splenic injuries.[12]

A magnetic resonance imaging (MRI) scan is rarely used in the initial evaluation of blunt abdominal trauma because of its excessive time requirement. The relative efficiency of CT makes MRI less useful for sport-related abdominal injuries.[12] Renal angiography may be beneficial in athletes with prolonged hematuria or reappearance of gross hematuria after a renal injury.[12]

SUMMARY

Sports medicine physicians should be aware of the many injuries that are associated with blunt abdominal trauma. From benign diaphragmatic spasms and rectus abdominis hematomas to more the concerning liver, splenic, renal, and pancreatic injuries, the sideline physician needs to be able to triage athletic-related injuries because patients can quickly deteriorate. Furthermore, many athletes will ask their physician about return-to-play recommendations following blunt abdominal trauma. Although little written return-to-play guidelines exist, the sports medicine physician should have a working knowledge of the pathophysiology of various abdominal injuries to best advise his or her team members.

REFERENCES

1. Bergqvist D, Hedelin H, Karlsson G, et al. Abdominal trauma during thirty years: analysis of a large case series. Injury 1981;13:93–9.
2. Hootman JM, Dick R, Agel J. Epidemiology of collegiate injuries for 15 sports: summary and recommendations for injury prevention initiatives. J Athl Train 2007;42(2):311–9.
3. Johnson R. Abdominal wall injuries: rectus abdominis strains, oblique strains, rectus sheath hematoma. Curr Sports Med Rep 2006;5:99–103.
4. Rifat S, Gilvydis R. Blunt abdominal trauma in sports. Curr Sports Med Rep 2003; 2:93–7.
5. Cherry WB, Mueller PS. Rectus sheath hematoma: review of 126 cases at a single institution. Medicine 2006;85(2):105–10.
6. Klingor PJ, Wetscher G, Glaser K, et al. The use of ultrasound to differentiate rectus sheath hematoma from other acute abdominal disorders. Surg Endosc 1999;13:1129–34.
7. Parmelee-Peters K, Moeller J. Liver trauma in a high school football player. Curr Sports Med Rep 2004;3:95–9.
8. Karam O, La Scala G, LeCoultre C, et al. Liver function tests in children with blunt abdominal traumas. Eur J Pediatr Surg 2007;17:313–6.
9. Puranik SR, Hayes JS, Long J, et al. Liver enzymes as a predictor of liver damage due to blunt abdominal trauma in children. South Med J 2002;95:203–6.

10. Gannon EH, Howard T. Splenic injuries in athletes: a review. Curr Sports Med Rep 2010;9(2):111–4.
11. Geddes R, Irish K. Boarder belly: splenic injuries resulting from ski and snowboarding accidents. Emerg Med Australas 2005;17:157–62.
12. Walter KD. Radiographic evaluation of the patient with sport-related abdominal trauma. Curr Sports Med Rep 2007;6:115–9.
13. Miller KS, Mcaninch JW. Radiographic assessment of renal trauma: our 15-year experience. J Urol 1995;154:352–5.
14. Holmes FC, Hunt JJ, Sevier TL. Renal injury in sport. Curr Sports Med Rep 2003; 2:103–9.
15. Bernard J. Renal trauma: evaluation, management, and return to play. Curr Sports Med Rep 2009;8(2):98–103.
16. Echlin PS, Klein WB. Pancreatic injury in the athlete. Curr Sports Med Rep 2005;4: 96–101.
17. Diercks DB, Mehrotra A, Nazarian DJ, et al. Clinical policy: critical issues in the evaluation of adult patients presenting to the emergency department with acute blunt abdominal trauma. Ann Emerg Med 2011;57(4):387–404.
18. Coley BD, Mutabagani KH, Martin LC, et al. Focused abdominal sonography for trauma (FAST) in children with abdominal trauma. J Trauma 2000;48:902–6.

Closed Kidney Injury

Tracey A. Viola, DO

KEYWORDS

- Blunt renal trauma • Kidney • Trauma • Injury • AAST organ injury scale

KEY POINTS

- The kidney is the most common urologic organ injured.
- Most renal injuries are due to blunt trauma.
- Patient history, examination, and imaging studies will guide management decisions.
- The American Association for the Surgery of Trauma has developed an Organ Injury Severity scale, which correlates with computed tomography scan findings.
- Most renal injuries can be managed nonoperatively.

INTRODUCTION

It has been estimated that, every year, children under the age of 18 account for 30 million emergency room visits, and 7.5 million of these are due to trauma.[1] Trauma is the leading cause of death in children.[2,3] The most common causes of trauma in pediatrics are falls and motor vehicle accidents (MVA).[1,4,5]

The prevalence of renal injury in blunt trauma ranges from 1%,[6] 1.4% to 3.25%,[7] 10%,[8] and 10% to 20%,[5] and the kidney is the most common urologic injury.[8-11] Between 80% and 90% of all renal injuries are due to a blunt mechanism,[6-8] and in children 90% are caused by blunt trauma.[4,5] With a blunt injury, either the ribs or the abdominal organs hit the kidneys.[7] Most isolated renal injuries, 95% to 98%, are minor and conservatively treated. Penetrating injuries make up 10% to 20% of injuries and are typically a gunshot or stab wound.[8] The focus of this article is on closed renal injury; therefore, penetrating injury is not discussed.

Epidemiology of renal injury has been described from retrospective reviews. In an analysis of the National Trauma Data Bank, from 1994 to 2003, Kuan and coworkers found that boys and men account for 73.8% of renal injuries, and 74.2% of these are in people less than 40 years old.[6] Santucci and colleauges' consensus statement

Disclosures: None.
Conflicts of Interest: None.
Family Practice and Sports Medicine, Lake Placid Health Center, 29 Church Street, Lake Placid, NY 12946, USA
E-mail address: tracey.viola@gmail.com

Clin Sports Med 32 (2013) 219–227
http://dx.doi.org/10.1016/j.csm.2012.12.002

estimates the mean age is 20 to 30 years.[7] In adults, MVA is the most common cause of renal injury.[5,8]

In regard to sports, both organized and recreational, contact and noncontact, sports have been associated with renal injury, although injury is rare overall. Almost all sports-related injuries are blunt[11] and are caused by blunt abdominal or flank injury, rapid deceleration, or high-velocity impacts caused either by objects that are part of the sport or by high-speed sports.[5]

Wan and colleagues[12] looked at the National Pediatric Trauma Registry from 1990 to 1999 and described injuries related to contact sports. Of a total of 81,923 trauma cases, only 5439 (6.64%) were due to sports in school-age children, and only 459 were abdominal or testicular (0.56% of all reported) injury. No injury resulted in functional loss of kidney. Although 62% of kidney injuries were related to football, other sports included baseball, basketball, hockey, and soccer. McAleer and colleagues[13] reviewed their trauma registry from July 1984 through December 2000 and found only 6 renal injuries were caused by team sports. Rates of renal injury were as follows, in decreasing frequency: bicycling (27.6%), falls (23.5%), all-terrain vehicle riding (8.2%), playground (8.2%), motorcycling (6.1%), team sports (6.1%), skateboarding (6.1%), rollerblading (6.1%), playing ball (4.1%), equestrian sports (3.1%), and trampoline jumping (1%). No kidneys were lost in this series. Wu and Gaines report similar findings from another pediatric trauma database, in which contact and organized sports had less significant renal injury than dirt bikes, all-terrain-vehicle rollovers and riding, and bicycles.[14]

Many of the trauma databases are descriptive of urban populations, so Lloyd and colleagues[15] studied adults at the Vail Valley Medical Center, Vail, CO. They specifically excluded MVAs and found that 85% of renal injuries were related to snow sports. These patients had different injury patterns than previously described in the urban population, fewer associated injuries, and less hypotension.

Management options in renal trauma are based on history and mechanism of injury, examination findings (hematuria, vitals, other injuries), and imaging, with the goal to determine who can be managed nonoperatively versus who needs surgical intervention, for preservation of life and renal function, with minimal morbidity.

PATIENT HISTORY

As described earlier, the most common mechanism for renal injury is blunt trauma. The kidney is protected posteriorly by the ribs and back muscles, and anteriorly by the abdominal organs.[7] Rapid deceleration injuries, for example, a fall or MVA, can also be significant because the renal hilum (pedicle and pyleoureteral junction) is fixed, and great forces are transmitted through this fixed area,[4,7,9] with risk of vascular and uteropelvic junction injuries.[4,7] Therefore, the history of the injury is important in risk-stratifying patients.

Another important factor in the history of injury is the age of the patient. There is thought that children are more likely to sustain renal trauma than their adult counterparts. Explanations such as greater size of kidney compared with the body, less perirenal fat to cushion the kidney, weaker abdominal muscles, and less protection from ribs, resulting in transmission of greater forces, have been postulated.[2,4,5,7] In a retrospective review of 34 pediatric and 35 adult blunt renal trauma victims, Brown and coworkers found that although children were more likely to sustain major (grade IV or V) renal injury, they had lower overall injury severity scores (a scale that describes multiple injuries). The most common mechanism of injury in children was falls (44%), and in adults the most common mechanism of injury was MVA (80%) in this series.[2]

PHYSICAL EXAMINATION

In the triage of any trauma patient, initial assessment should include the ABCs (airway, breathing, and circulation with pulse and blood pressure measurements). Hemodynamic instability in children or adults, not responsive to resuscitation efforts, should be surgically explored (**Fig. 1** shows the assessment algorithm).[4,5,9] If the patient is stable, a secondary survey should be performed next. Of note, whereas in adults blood pressure is an adequate assessment of volume status,[4] in children, it is not, as they can be normotensive and hypovolemic.[4,5]

On examination, special attention should be paid to signs that indicate a renal injury. Objective signs include gross hematuria,[4,5] flank hematoma,[5,7,9] flank[5,7,16] or abdominal eccymoses[4] or tenderness,[4,5,9,16] pelvic pain,[4] rib fractures or pain,[4,5,7,9,16] transverse process pain,[16] penetrating injuries,[5,9] or abdominal examination with peritoneal signs (rebound tenderness, guarding).[16]

After examination, urinalysis should be performed.[5,16] The most common laboratory finding is microscopic hematuria,[5] and 80% to 95% of significant renal injuries in adults do present with hematuria.[7,8] If microscopic hematuria is present, quantification can help determine if further imaging is indicated. Predictors of significant renal injury in adults include microscopic hematuria and hypotension,[5,7,9] and in children predictors of significant renal injury include greater than 50 red blood cells (RBCs) per high-power field and should be further imaged.[4,5,7] Of importance, the presence or absence and number of RBCs do not necessarily correlate to injury.[4,7,9] For example, with a deceleration injury, there may not be hematuria despite pedicle injuries.[9] If gross hematuria is noted, further imaging should be performed.[5,16]

Additional laboratory evaluation should include complete blood count, complete chemistry including electrolytes, creatinine, glucose, liver function tests, amylase, and lipase[5,16] to evaluate for other abdominal organ injury. Radiographs can be helpful in the evaluation of rib and transverse process fractures.[16]

Serial examinations, including vital signs, abdominal examinations, and hematocrit, are also important in the ongoing care of renal injury.[4,5] If no imaging is necessary, Santucci and colleagues[7] recommend observation and a follow-up urinalysis in 3 weeks.

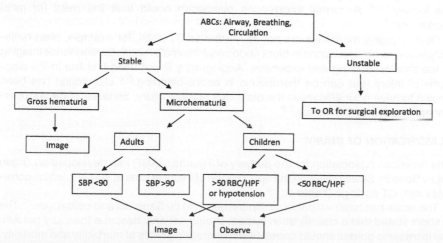

Fig. 1. Triage of blunt renal trauma.

IMAGING AND ADDITIONAL TESTING

As noted earlier, patients with gross hematuria should be imaged, as well as adults with microscopic hematuria and systolic blood pressure less than 90, and children with more than 50 RBC per high-power field or hypotension. In addition to these criteria, mechanism of injury should be taken into account, and any significant injury, such as a deceleration or high-speed injury, should be imaged.[4,7]

Testing these criteria, in children with the findings listed above (>50 RBC per high-power field, hypotension, or mechanism of injury [MOI]) who are imaged, a significant injury will not be missed.[5] In adults, if gross hematuria, hypotension, and a significant MOI are absent, imaging is not necessary.[9] However, in contrast to the urban data in trauma registries, the series of patients from Vail, CO (a rural area), if imaging were restricted to gross hematuria or microscopic hematuria and hypotension, 23% of grade 2 to 4 injuries would have been missed.[15] Future studies must be performed in rural settings to confirm or deny that they need different imaging criteria.

The gold standard in imaging of blunt abdominal trauma is the computed tomography (CT) scan with intravascular (IV) contrast,[5,9] because it gives reliable information on the abdominal cavity and retroperitoneal structures[4] and is readily available, rapid, and accurate for diagnosing and staging renal injuries and other organ injuries.[7-9] For assessing renal trauma, a renal protocol CT should be performed, consisting first of noncontrast images, to see the renal vasculature[4] and acute bleeding and hematoma formation,[8] but will miss collecting system injuries. A medial hematoma on these images suggests a renal pedicle injury.[9] Then IV contrast is injected, and a set of images is obtained for parenchymal definition, followed by delayed images to visualize the collecting system.[4,8] On postcontrast images, lack of parenchymal contrast on the early phase images suggests arterial injury, and medial extravasation on delayed films correlates to pedicle injury or ureteropelvic junction disruption.[9]

Hom studied the rate of intra-abdominal injury after a negative CT with IV contrast in 2596 pediatric patients and found the negative predictive value of CT was 99.8% and the rate of injury despite negative CT was 0.19%. Of these patients, only 5 needed further intervention, and only 2 of these were due to renal injury.[1] If immediate operative treatment is necessary, for example, where patients are unstable, a one-shot intravenous pyelogram can be performed, with an IV contrast bolus of 2 mL/kg, and follow-up plain radiograph. The purpose of this study is to document the function of the kidney.[4,7-9] A normal intravenous pyelogram could limit the need for renal exploration.[7]

Other imaging modalities are not as reliable as CT scan, for example, plain radiographs are rarely used alone in blunt abdominal trauma[8]; magnetic resonance imaging is too time consuming and expensive. Angiography is not used first line in the diagnosis of injury, but can be therapeutic in active bleeding.[7-9] Ultrasound has been shown to have poor efficacy in the diagnosis of renal injury, because of the retroperitoneal location of the kidney.[7,9]

CLASSIFICATION OF INJURY

The American Association for the Surgery of Trauma (AAST) has developed an Organ Injury Severity Scale based on the appearance of injury at time of surgery, which correlates with CT findings (**Table 1**).[7-9]

This scale has been validated multiple times, first by Santucci and colleagues.[17] The authors stated that a classification system should not only describe the injury but also the increasing grades should correlate with increasing rates of morbidity and mortality. In their retrospective review of 2467 patients, they found AAST grades have

Table 1
AAST organ injury severity scale
Grade I	Contusion OR subcapsular hematoma, nonexpanding
Grade II	Cortical renal laceration less than 1 cm without urinary extravasation OR retroperitoneal perirenal hematoma, nonexpanding
Grade III	Laceration extending to medulla, greater than 1 cm, without extravasation
Grade IV	Laceration extending through collecting system with extravasation, OR vascular injury or segmental infarction without avulsion of the hilum and contained hematoma
Grade V	Shattered or fractured kidney (multiple grade IV lacerations) OR vascular injury with hilar avulsion and devascularization

a statistically significant correlation with the need for surgery (15 times greater risk per grade increase) and nephrectomy (7 times per grade increase) (**Table 2**). Kuan and colleagues[6] did a second validation study and found that higher AAST grade was associated with higher rates of morbidity as measured by nephrectomy and dialysis, and mortality.

MANAGEMENT/OUTCOMES

The goal in the management of renal injuries is to preserve life and renal function[8,18] and minimize morbidity,[18] such as hemorrhage, and local and systemic infection.[8] Most injuries are grade I contusions and can be managed with supportive care.[5] The goal of treatment is to prevent morbidity (hemorrhage, abnormal renal function, decrease costs and hospitalization rates) and mortality.[19] Most blunt trauma is managed without surgery, in part because of the accuracy of CT grading, from grade I to IV.[5] In a systematic review by Santucci, there was literature support for a trial of conservative management, in the absence of hemodynamic instability and renal pelvis or vascular injury, for grades I to IV.[17] In a retrospective review of 55 children with renal injury, 87% were managed conservatively, and all grades I to III (65% of all injuries) were nonoperative. Twenty-nine percent of grade IV and 60% of grade V injuries needed surgical treatment. Grade IV and V injuries took longer to clear gross hematuria.[10]

In the world of sports medicine, a frequent question is, when can an injured player return to sports? Although there is no absolute consensus, the suggested algorithm is bed rest until resolution of gross hematuria[10,19,20] and then return to full activity when microscopic hematuria has resolved. With minor injury, this can take 2 to 6 weeks, but with more severe injury, may take 6 to 12 months.[5] In a retrospective review of National Football League renal injuries from 1986 to 2004, Brophy and colleagues[16] identified 52 cases, with the most common injury being contusion (81%, 15.1 average

Table 2		
Risk of surgical treatment or nephrectomy by AAST grade of injury		
AAST Grade	**Surgical Treatment**	**Nephrectomy**
I	0%	0%
II	15%	0%
III	76%	3%
IV	78%	9%
V	93%	86%

days missed), laceration (11%, 59.8 days missed), and stones and "dysfunction" (8%, 14 days missed). Ninety-four percent of injuries were contact related; none required surgery, and all returned to play.

SURGICAL INDICATIONS

It is well agreed on that hemodynamic instability is an absolute criteria for surgical treatment.[5,7,8,17,19] Probable indications for surgical exploration include the following: expanding renal mass, large pulsating perirenal hematoma indicating pedicle avulsion,[7,8,17,19] ureteral injury or extracapsular urinary extravasation, and renal pelvis injury.[8,17,19] Relative indications are as follows: shattered kidney, urinary extravasation with devitalized segment,[19] poor staging,[8,17,19] associated intra-abdominal injury,[5,17,19] significant arterial injury,[17] and gross fragmentation or tissue destruction, as devascularized segments have higher rates of complications.[7,8,17] With a vascular injury, more than 2 hours of ischemia results in irreversible damage.[7] Surgical techniques are beyond the scope of this article, but of interest, Yeung and Brandes surveyed trauma surgeons and urologists regarding their surgical practices, and there is no consensus between the groups on some of their management guidelines.[21]

FOLLOW-UP IMAGING

Regarding follow-up imaging, it is agreed on that grade I and II renal injuries do not need follow-up imaging and is likely not necessary in nonoperative grade III injuries[7,8,22] and IV without urinary extravasation.[7,8] In a review of the Los Angeles County and University of Southern California Trauma registry, no patients with a grade I to III renal injury managed nonoperatively developed any complication.[20] Grade IV injuries with urinary extravasation and grade V should be monitored with repeat imaging in 36 to 72 hours.[7,8,22] In a study by Malcolm and colleagues,[22] on conservatively managed patients, 84% had follow-up imaging 24 to 48 hours after admission, and there were no complications in those not re-imaged (they were all grade I-III). If they had only re-imaged grade IV injuries with extravasation and grade V, they would have had a cost reduction of 94% (**Table 3**). Any worsening of patient status, such as hemodynamic instability, fever, or examination findings, should be re-imaged.[7,8,20] The goal of follow-up imaging is to identify complications, such as worsening urinary extravasation, ongoing hemorrhage, and pseudoaneurysm.[7,20]

PREDICTORS OF FAILURE

In a 5-year retrospective review by Simmons and coworkers, 88% of their patients were initially managed nonoperatively, and of these, 4.1% later required intervention. Of those that failed conservative management, they had higher injury severity scores (were more seriously injured), had worse acidosis, needed more blood products, and had longer hospital stays.[23] Similarly, McGuire and colleagues looked at injuries grades III to V and performed logistic regression models. On multivariate analysis of those managed with initial operative treatment, grade V injury and need for platelet transfusion predicted the need for surgical intervention. Of those managed conservatively, older age and hypotension predicted who would have complications.[18]

COMPLICATIONS

Acute complications of renal trauma include urinary extravasation (80%–90% will resolve spontaneously),[7] expansion of urinoma[4,7,8] or hematoma, urinary tract infection, ileus, and pain.[4] Less acutely, but within the first month of injury, complications

Table 3		
Management based on AAST staging after initial CT		
AAST Grade	Immediate Treatment	CT Results
I	No gross hematuria: Outpatient management, no routine imaging	N/A
	Gross hematuria: Bed rest until gross hematuria resolves, observation, no routine imaging	N/A
II	Admit for observation, no routine imaging	N/A
III	Admit for observation, no routine imaging	N/A
IV	No urinary extravasation: no routine imaging	N/A
	Urinary extravasation: Repeat CT at 48 h	CT stable: monitor Arterial bleed: consider angiography Urinary extravasation: consider stent vs drain
V	Repeat CT at 48 h	CT stable: monitor Arterial bleed: consider angiography Urinary extravasation: consider stent vs drain

include perinephric abscess,[7,8] sepsis,[8] delayed hemorrhage due to arteriovenous fistula, or pseudoaneurysm.[7,8] Chronic complications include abnormal or loss of renal function,[4,7] Page kidney (hypertension due to constrictive ischemic nephropathy due to mass effect of large subcapsular hematoma),[4,7,8] arteriovenous malformations, fistula,[4] hypertension, hydronephrosis, calculus formation, and chronic pyelonephritis.[8]

SPECIAL CIRCUMSTANCES

The American Academy of Pediatrics Committee on Sports Medicine and Fitness has recommended those with a solitary kidney be given a "qualified yes" on an individual case-by-case basis involving appropriate counseling for contact, collision, and limited-contact sports.[5] In the Preparticipation Physical Evaluation Monograph, protective measures, such as a flak jacket and discussion of long-term consequencesand treatment of injuries, are recommended as part of this informed consent process.[5,24] In addition, in Santucci and colleagues[7] consensus statement, it is noted that pre-existing renal abnormalities pose a higher risk to kidneys, and in the Preparticipation Physical Evaluation Monograph there is mention of abnormalities such as the pelvic, iliac or multicystic kidney, hydronephrosis, and ureteropelvic junction abnormalities with consideration of not allowing participation.[24] Although loss of a solitary kidney is certainly catastrophic, an article by Psooy does an excellent job to put risk in perspective. She notes that sports that carry a risk to renal injury have 5 times the risk of a head injury, yet having only 1 brain does not deter participation in sports. For children who have higher risk of renal injury, whether due to a solitary or an abnormal kidney, counseling of the patient (and parents) is important and should include information on protective equipment (rib protectors, blocking vest, kidney belt, although there are no existing data on efficacy), and long-term consequences, such as risk of renal insufficiency, dialysis, or transplant. Last, the higher risk sports include bicycling, sledding, skiing, snowboarding, and horseback riding; however, MVA is more common than all of these.[25]

SUMMARY

Renal injury is uncommon, and the prevalence of renal injury in sports is rare. The risk of loss of a kidney in sports is exceedingly rare, and this should help guide the Sports Medicine physician in clearance of an athlete with a solitary kidney or congenital abnormality. The history of mechanism of injury, examination findings, laboratory tests, and imaging studies guide management decisions to surgical intervention or conservative treatment. CT is the gold standard for the diagnosis of renal injury in the stable patient. The American Association for the Surgery of Trauma Organ Injury Severity scale is a reliable tool for management decisions and correlates with morbidity.

REFERENCES

1. Hom J. The risk of intra-abdominal injuries in pediatric patients with stable blunt abdominal trauma and negative abdominal computed tomography. Acad Emerg Med 2010;17(5):469–75.
2. Brown SL, Elder JS, Spirnak JP. Are pediatric patients more susceptible to major renal injury from blunt trauma? A comparative study. J Urol 1998;160:138–40.
3. Fraser JD, Aguayo P, Ostlie DJ, et al. Review of the evidence on the management of blunt renal trauma in pediatric patients. Pediatr Surg Int 2009;25(2):125–32.
4. Buckley JC, McAninch JW. The diagnosis, management and outcomes of pediatric renal injuries. Urol Clin North Am 2006;33:33–40.
5. Bernard JJ. Renal trauma: evaluation, management, and return to play. Curr Sports Med Rep 2009;8(2):98–103.
6. Kuan JK, Wright JL, Nathens AB, et al. American Association for the Surgery of Trauma Organ Injury Scale for kidney injuries predicts nephrectomy, dialysis, and death in patients with blunt injury and nephrectomy for penetrating injuries. J Trauma 2006;60(2):351–6.
7. Santucci RA, Wessells H, Bartsch G, et al. Evaluation and management of renal injuries: consensus statement of the renal trauma subcommittee. BJU Int 2004; 93(7):937–54.
8. Alonso RC, Nacenta SB, Martinez PD, et al. Kidney in danger: CT findings of blunt and penetrating renal trauma. Radiographics 2009;29(7):2033–53.
9. Alsikafi NF, Rosenstein DI. Staging, evaluation, and nonoperative management of renal injuries. Urol Clin North Am 2006;33(1):13–9.
10. Margenthaler JA, Weber TR, Keller MS. Blunt renal trauma in children: experience with conservative management at a pediatric trauma center. J Trauma 2002; 52(5):928–32.
11. Styn NR, Wan J. Urologic sports injuries in children. Curr Urol Rep 2010;11(2): 114–21.
12. Wan J, Corvino TF, Greenfield SP, et al. Kidney and testicle injury in team and individual sports: data from the national pediatric trauma registry. J Urol 2003;170: 1528–31.
13. McAleer IM, Kaplan GW, LoSasso BE. Renal and testis injuries in team sports. J Urol 2002;168:1805–7.
14. Wu HY, Gaines BA. Dirt bikes and all terrain vehicles: the real threat to pediatric kidneys. J Urol 2007;178(4):1672–4.

15. Lloyd GL, Slack S, McWilliams KL, et al. Renal trauma from recreational accidents manifests different injury patterns than urban renal trauma. J Urol 2012;188(1): 163–8.
16. Brophy RH, Gamradt SC, Barnes RP, et al. Kidney injuries in professional American football. Am J Sports Med 2008;36:85–90.
17. Santucci RA, McAninch JW, Safir MS, et al. Validation of the American Association for the Surgery of Trauma organ injury severity scale for the kidney. J Trauma 2001;50:195–200.
18. McGuire J, Bultitude MF, Davis P, et al. Predictors of outcome for blunt high grade renal injury treated with conservative intent. J Urol 2011;185(1):187–91.
19. Santucci RA, Fisher MB. The literature increasingly supports expectant (conservative) management of renal trauma–a systematic review. J Trauma 2005;59(2): 493–503.
20. Bukur M, Inaba K, Barmparas G, et al. Routine follow-up imaging of kidney injuries may not be justified. J Trauma 2011;70(5):1229–33.
21. Yeung LL, Brandes SB. Contemporary management of renal trauma: differences between urologists and trauma surgeons. J Trauma Acute Care Surg 2012;72(1): 68–75.
22. Malcolm JB, Derweesh IH, Mehrazin R, et al. Nonoperative management of blunt renal trauma: is routine early follow-up imaging necessary? BMC Urol 2008;8: 11–6.
23. Simmons JD, Haraway AN, Schmieg RE Jr, et al. Blunt renal trauma and the predictors of failure of non-operative management. J Miss State Med Assoc 2010;51(5):131–3.
24. Preparticipation Physical Evaluation. 4th edition. Bernhardt D, Roberts W, editors. American Academy of Pediatrics. Elk Grove, IL. 2010.
25. Psooy K. Sports and the solitary kidney: how to counsel parents. Can J Urol 2006; 13(3):3120–6.

Closed Liver Injury

Deena C. Casiero, MD[a,b,c,d,e],*

KEYWORDS

- Blunt abdominal trauma • Closed liver injury • Nonoperative management
- Liver injury grading scale • Diagnostic imaging • Return-to-play guidelines

KEY POINTS

- The liver is the most commonly injured organ in blunt abdominal trauma.
- Physical examination findings may be subtle or absent in patients with underlying liver injury.
- CT is the test of choice in hemodynamically stable patients.
- Liver injuries are graded I–VI as identified on CT scan or at the time of surgery.
- Higher grades of injury are associated with higher morbidity and mortality.
- Hemodynamically stable patients, regardless of grade of injury, are generally treated nonoperatively with close observation in a monitored setting.
- Unstable patients usually undergo urgent laparotomy.
- There has been a paradigm shift toward nonoperative management in hemodynamically stable patients, which has led to a decrease in mortality in these patients.
- Return-to-play guidelines do not exist for patients who suffered a closed liver injury.

INTRODUCTION

Abdominal trauma is a rare but potentially fatal occurrence in sports-related activity. Up to 10% of reported abdominal injuries are caused by trauma during athletic events.[1,2] The liver is the most commonly injured organ in blunt abdominal trauma.[3] Contact and collision sports, such as rugby, soccer, and football, account for most closed liver injuries caused by direct trauma to the abdomen.[1,2] Noncontact sports, such as skiing and snowboarding, can cause liver trauma secondary to a deceleration mechanism.[2]

Most closed liver injuries are minor and can be treated nonoperatively with observation alone or with adjunctive treatment using arteriography and embolization of

Disclosures: None.
[a] ProHEALTH Care Associates, 2800 Marcus Avenue, Lake Success, NY 11042, USA; [b] USA Seven's Women's Rugby, Arapahoe Avenue Boulder, Colorado 80302, USA; [c] Hofstra University, Fulton Avenue, Hempstead, NY 11549, USA; [d] US Open Tennis Championships, Flushing Meadow, Corona Park Road, Flushing, NY, USA; [e] New York Islanders, Hempstead Turnpike, Uniondale, NY 11553, USA
* 2800 Marcus Avenue, Suite 102 Lake Success, NY 11042, USA.
E-mail address: Dcasiero@prohealthcare.com

Clin Sports Med 32 (2013) 229–238
http://dx.doi.org/10.1016/j.csm.2012.12.007
0278-5919/13/$ – see front matter © 2013 Elsevier Inc. All rights reserved.

sportsmed.theclinics.com

bleeding vessels.[3–15] As few as 10% to 14% of patients with liver injuries require operative intervention due to hemodynamic instability or failure of nonoperative management.[7,16] Because of the potentially fatal nature of some closed liver injuries, it is imperative that sports medicine physicians be adept at evaluating and appropriately triaging these injuries. The goal of this article is to review the mechanisms of injury, signs, symptoms and the appropriate referral of potentially fatal closed liver injuries.

MECHANISM OF INJURY

There are several pathophysiologic mechanisms that can occur during sports-related trauma that may result in closed liver injury. The application of blunt forces exerted against the anterior abdominal wall can cause compression of the underlying viscera against the posterior thoracic wall or the vertebral column. This can result in crush injuries that cause subcapsular or intraparenchymal hematomas in the underlying liver.[1,17] Sports that involve high-intensity acceleration and deceleration forces can cause lacerations of the liver at its points of attachment to the peritoneum or stretch injuries to the intima and media of nearby arteries.[1,17]

SIDELINE EVALUATION

Sports medicine physicians on the sidelines of athletic events may be charged with trying to discern benign abdominal wall injuries from potentially fatal closed liver trauma. This is a challenging task because most severe abdominal injuries have a subtle initial presentation. In most cases, the definitive diagnosis can only be made in the emergency room or with advanced imaging. The decision to allow athletes to return to play versus removed from the competition and transported to a hospital for further evaluation, however, is in the hands of sports medicine physicians, highlighting the importance of the sideline physician's comfort level with evaluation and management of closed liver injuries (**Box 1**).

As with most athletic injuries, the mechanism of injury, history, and physical examination are essential parts of the diagnostic puzzle.

HISTORY

- Was it a direct blow to the abdomen?
- Was it a deceleration mechanism?
- Where is the pain? (right upper quadrant, right chest wall, right flank pain, or right shoulder/neck pain due to radiating pain from diaphragmatic irritation)
- Did it start immediately or develop slowly over time?
- Is it focal or generalized? (Localized abdominal pain can occur with abdominal wall injury whereas generalized abdominal pain is more concerning for underlying organ damage because of the peritoneal irritation that may occur.)
- Any associated symptoms? (nausea, vomiting, altered sensorium)

PHYSICAL EXAMINATION

- Unfortunately, the initial presentation of a patient with severe liver injury can range from a conscious patient with subtle complaints and normal vital signs to one that is obtunded and in a state of severe shock.
- The most common findings are abdominal tenderness coupled with peritoneal signs, but these findings are not sensitive or specific for liver injury.
- The accuracy of the physical examination has been reported to be as low as 55% to 65% in identifying abdominal trauma.[18]

Box 1
Sideline evaluation

History

Mechanism of injury

  Direct blow

  Deceleration mechanism

Location and severity of pain

  Right upper quadrant

  Right chest wall

  Right flank

Associated symptoms

  Nausea

  Vomiting

  Altered sensorium

Physical examination

ABCDEs

Abdominal tenderness

Peritoneal signs

  Guarding

  Rebound tenderness

  Rigidity

Cullen sign

Check for associated injuries

Abbreviation: ABCDEs, Airway, Breathing, Circulation, Disability, Exposure.

- Peritoneal signs include abdominal guarding, rebound tenderness, or rigidity.
- An athlete's report of pain or discomfort with laughing, jumping, or coughing can be a sign of peritoneal irritation.
- The presence of Cullen sign (a periumbilical hematoma) may suggest hemoperitoneum.

ASSOCIATED INJURIES

When evaluating athletes with blunt abdominal trauma, it is imperative to consider associated injuries. One recent study showed that 80% of patients with hepatic trauma had at least one concomitant injury.[8] Examples of other injuries that are commonly associated with liver injury are spleen injuries, lower rib fractures, pelvic fractures, and spinal cord injury.

INITIAL EVALUATION AND MANAGEMENT

The sideline physician must always keep in mind that the absence of physical findings does not preclude an underlying liver injury and that no sign exists that is exclusively diagnostic of a liver injury.[19–21] Therefore, a thorough and comprehensive evaluation is needed to ensure that a closed liver injury is not missed. The initial evaluation should always start with the primary survey: airway, breathing, circulation, disability (neurologic status), and exposure. If, based on the primary assessment, a patient is found hemodynamically unstable, the patient should be transported to the hospital immediately for continued evaluation and treatment. Details regarding the treatment of the hemodynamically unstable patient with liver trauma are beyond the scope of this article.

In the cases of hemodynamically stable patients with suspected liver injury, many studies concur that diagnostic imaging confirming the diagnosis and close observation in a monitored setting are the standard of care.[3–5,7–14]

DIAGNOSTIC EVALUATION
CT

In hemodynamically stable patients with suspected closed liver injury, many studies suggest that CT is the test of choice.[1,11,12,14,22,23] It has been shown to be more sensitive than ultrasound in addition to demonstrating greater anatomic detail, which can result in more accurate injury grading and diagnosis.[1,22] The improvements in speed and availability of CT over the past few decades have made this test an important one in the evaluation of any hemodynamically stable trauma victim.[24,25]

The benefits of CT include
- Noninvasive testing
- Demonstrating good anatomic definition
- Possibly detecting presence as well as source of hemoperitoneum
- Allowing for evaluation of associated injuries (eg, head spinal column, chest, and pelvis)

The disadvantages of CT include
- Radiation exposure
- Intravenous contrast needed (oral contrast not needed because it does not usually add to accuracy of diagnosis and usually delays imaging)[11,22]
- Relatively high cost compared with ultrasound
- Cannot be used in hemodynamically unstable patients[26]

Ultrasound

The bedside use of ultrasound has long been a part of the evaluation of trauma patients, especially those who are hemodynamically unstable. It has largely been replaced by CT, however, in those patients who are stable enough to undergo the gold standard test.

The benefits of ultrasound include
- Fast
- Portable
- Cost-effective
- Noninvasiveness (as opposed to diagnostic peritoneal lavage)

The disadvantages of ultrasound include
- Low sensitivity (85%)[22]
- Operator dependent[27]
- Can identify intraperitoneal fluid but sometimes misses solid organ injuries[22]

Diagnostic Peritoneal Lavage

The role of diagnostic peritoneal lavage in the evaluation of trauma patients has been on the decline for many years. It had played an integral role since its introduction in the

1960s but the advances in CT and ultrasound have forced it out of favor especially in regards to those patients who are stable enough to undergo the more advanced tests. DPL can accurately determine the presence of blood within the peritoneum of hemodynamically unstable patients and for this reason the test is still in use today.[28]

Advantages of DPL
- Triage of unstable patients
- Can detect small amount of intraperitoneal blood

Disadvantages of DPL
- Risk of infection
- Risk of intraperitoneal injury
- False-positive results or small amount of blood found in peritoneum may lead to unnecessary laparotomy in otherwise stable patients who could be treated nonoperatively

Other Imaging

Plain radiographs are not used for the specific diagnosis of liver trauma.[22] They are nonspecific but can be helpful if a rib fracture is identified, which may increase the suspicion for liver injury. MRI is also of limited value because the test is time consuming. There may be a subset of patients, however, who cannot undergo CT scans or who are allergic to intravenous contrast that may benefit from an MRI. Angiography is a time-consuming procedure that is generally reserved for patients who are hemodynamically stable and require embolization of bleeding vessels.[11,15]

GRADING OF LIVER INJURIES

The American Association for the Surgery of Trauma developed a hepatic organ injury scale that is used to grade the severity of liver injuries (**Table 1**).[16] This grading system is used as a tool to help clinicians determine the likelihood of success with

Table 1 Hepatic organ injury scale		
Grade	**Type**	**Description**
I	Hematoma	Subcapsular, <10% of surface area
	Laceration	Capsular tear, <1 cm parenchymal depth
II	Hematoma	Subcapsular, 10%–50% surface area; or intraparenchymal <10 cm in diameter
	Laceration	Capsular tear 1–3 cm parenchymal depth <10 cm in length
III	Hematoma	Subcapsular, >50% surface area of ruptured subcapsular or parenchymal hematoma; intraparenchymal hematoma >10 cm or expanding
	Laceration	>3 cm Parenchymal depth
IV	Laceration	Parenchymal disruption involving 25%–75% of hepatic lobe or 1–3 Couinaud segments
V	Hematoma	Parenchymal disruption involving >75% of hepatic lobe or >3 Couinaud segments within a single lobe
	Vascular	Juxtahepatic venous injuries
VI	Vascular	Hepatic avulsion

Data from Tinkoff G, Esposito TJ, Reed J, et al. American Association for the surgery of Trauma Organ Injury Scale 1: spleen, liver and kidney, validation based on the National Trauma Data Bank. J Coll Surg 2008;207:646.

nonoperative management. Liver injuries given a grade of I, II, or III are more likely to be treated successfully with nonoperative management than injuries labeled as grade IV or V.[4,12,14,16] In 2008, one study reported that 67% of liver injuries were grades I, II, or III.[16] Grade VI injuries are generally hemodynamically unstable and are, therefore, treated with immediate surgical intervention.

MANAGEMENT

Advances in the availability, speed, and sensitivity of imaging modalities coupled with the improvement in critical care monitoring have facilitated a shift from operative to nonoperative care for the majority of hepatic injuries. This paradigm shift has been associated with a decrease in morbidity and mortality.[3,5,29] Hemodynamic status and grade of injury in addition to the presence of associated injuries are all taken into consideration when management decisions are made regarding operative versus nonoperative treatment.

NONOPERATIVE MANAGEMENT

Hemodynamically stable patients with blunt liver trauma can be treated with observation and the adjunctive use of arteriography and embolization when needed. Studies have shown greater than 90% success rates with this management strategy.[4,10,14,30] When a nonoperative treatment plan is chosen, it is imperative that a solid support structure be in place in the event that surgical intervention is needed. The immediate availability of an operating room, ICU beds, blood bank support, surgeons, and interventional radiologists increases survival rates in patients who are initially chosen for nonoperative management but ultimately fail it. For this reason, most patients who do not immediately require surgery are monitored as inpatients until their injuries are stabilized.

Observation

Observation for patients with hemodynamically stable liver injuries generally occurs in a monitored unit where there is increased availability of nursing and medical staff. This setting is optimal in the event that an urgent procedure, such as arteriography, needs to take place. Although no official evidence-based guidelines for inpatient observation have been set, one study shows that once a patient has normal serial abdominal examinations and a stable hematocrit for greater than 24 hours, the patient can usually be safely discharged home despite the grade of injury.[13]

Hepatic Embolization

Hepatic embolization is used as part of nonoperative management to control bleeding that does not require laparotomy. This procedure is performed by an interventional radiologist with experience in celiac artery catheterization and embolization techniques. Success rates of the procedure vary depending largely on institution, technique, and operator skill. This procedure has begun to replace initial surgical management in some institutions.[2,15,31]

Risks and Benefits of Nonoperative Management

The biggest benefit to nonoperative management is the elimination of the risks involved in surgery. The literature reports that anywhere from 50% to 86% of liver injuries that go directly to surgery have already achieved spontaneous hemostasis at the time of surgery.[4,5,8,12] There is a higher risk of missing an associated intra-abdominal injury, however, when laparotomy is not performed.

There is controversy in the literature regarding the need for multiple blood transfusions and whether this is increased or decreased in the nonoperative treatment groups. Potential risks of repeated blood transfusion include transfusion-related acute lung injury and transfusion-related immune modulation. Recent studies, however, have shown no significant difference or even a reduction in transfusion rates in the nonoperative groups compared with those undergoing laparotomy.[12] Hepatic embolization as a part of nonoperative management has its own inherent risks, including hepatic necrosis, pseudoaneurysm formation at the access site, and allergic reaction to the contrast dye.[32]

Failure Rates in Nonoperative Management

The failure of nonoperative treatment in patients with closed liver injury is defined as the need for surgical intervention. This can occur in the patient who remains hemodynamically stable but requires continued volume expansion or in patients who become hemodynamically unstable. Fewer than 3.5% of appropriately selected patients fail nonoperative management.[11,31] There are also higher failure rates reported in patients with grade IV and V injuries compared with those with grades I to III.[32]

SURGICAL MANAGEMENT

In hemodynamically unstable patients, urgent laparoscopy is the treatment of choice and gives patients the best chance at survival.[6,31] The operative management of closed liver injury, however, is a challenge for even the most experienced trauma surgeon. The liver is a large vascular organ with a dual blood supply that poses many obstacles during surgery. Emergent surgical intervention involves damage control techniques that aim to temporarily control brisk bleeding to allow patients to be hemodynamically resuscitated.[3,6] The definitive operative treatment involves a variety of surgical techniques, which are beyond the scope of this article.

MORBIDITY AND MORTALITY FOR HEPATIC INJURY

Morbidity and mortality rates in closed liver injuries vary greatly depending on injury grade.[30,32] The shift toward nonoperative management has improved the overall mortality rates over the years to 10% to 42%. This reduction has been most evident in the higher injury grades (III–V), which were treated almost exclusively with surgery in the past.[32,33]

Complications are common when treating closed liver trauma and increase with the severity of the injury. One study showed a respective increase in complications to be 5%, 22%, and 52% in injuries graded III, IV, and V.[9] Complications occur in hepatic injuries graded I and II as well but with less frequency. Morbidity rates have been found higher in patients managed nonoperatively because of the associated complications that occur with treatment interventions and prolonged length of stay.[9]

FOLLOW-UP CARE AND RETURN-TO-PLAY GUIDELINES

No guidelines exist in regard to the care and follow-up for patients with closed liver injuries who are treated nonoperatively. Some recent data suggest that ordering serial follow-up CT scans is unnecessary unless patients show signs of deterioration.[2,14,22] Follow-up imaging that is ordered several months out from injury to document healing also remains controversial.

Recommendations regarding duration of bed rest and when it is safe to resume daily activities has also not been established in the literature. The common practice has been to avoid strenuous activity for several weeks for grades I to III hepatic injuries. Higher-grade injuries (IV and V) generally are kept out of activity for closer to 3 months. There have been no studies, however, published on this topic.[34]

One of the most daunting decisions that sports medicine physicians have to make after blunt abdominal liver injury is when to safely return athletes to play. Unfortunately, there are no published guidelines that make this decision an easy one.[1,2] Like most return-to-play decisions, many factors should be taken into account. These include awaiting anatomic and functional healing of the liver in addition to assessing an athlete's mental readiness. As discussed previously, serial imaging is controversial but athletes should have normal liver enzymes and laboratory evidence of normal liver function before returning to sport. Protective devices, such as flak jackets, have not been studied. An athlete's mental readiness to return to sport must also be considered because the evaluation, diagnosis, and treatment of these injuries can be frightening for athletes.

SUMMARY

Although liver trauma is rare in athletics, sports medicine physicians must be aware of the signs and symptoms of these injuries. If liver trauma is suspected, athletes should be immediately transferred to the hospital especially if they are hemodynamically unstable. Management decisions are usually based on the hemodynamic stability of a patient. Ultrasound and diagnostic peritoneal lavage are generally reserved for unstable patients who may need to be taken immediately to surgery if the results are positive for hemoperitoneum. CT is the gold standard for hemodynamically stable patients. There has been a paradigm shift over the past few decades toward nonoperative management of hemodynamically stable patients given the lower mortality rates in this patient population. Liver injuries are graded by severity (I–VI) and the higher grades are associated with higher overall morbidity and mortality rates. Because return to play guidelines do not exist for these types of injuries, sports medicine physicians should apply basic return to play principles when making these decisions.

REFERENCES

1. Rifat S, Rimas G. Blunt abdominal trauma in sports. Curr Sports Med Rep 2003; 2(2):93–7.
2. Parmelee-Peters K, Moeller JL. Liver trauma in a high school football player. Curr Sports Med Rep 2004;3(2):95–9.
3. Richardson JD, Franklin GA, Lukan JK. Evolution in the management of hepatic trauma: a 25-year perspective. Ann Surg 2000;232:324–30.
4. Croce MA, Fabian TC, Menke PG, et al. Nonoperative management of blunt hepatic trauma is the treatment of choice for hemodynamically stable patients. Results of a prospective trial. Ann Surg 1995;221:744–53.
5. Malhotra AK, Fabian TC, Croce MA. Blunt hepatic injury: a paradigm shift from operative to nonoperative management in the 1990s. Ann Surg 2000;231:804–13.
6. Fabian TC, Croce MA, Stanford GG, et al. Factors affecting morbidity following hepatic trauma. A prospective analysis of 482 injuries. Ann Surg 1991;213:540–7.
7. Haller JA Jr, Papa P, Drugas G, et al. Nonoperative management of solid organ injuries in children. Is it safe? Ann Surg 1994;219:625–8.
8. Sanchez-Bueno F, Fernandez-Carrion J, Torres-Salmeron G, et al. Changes in diagnosis and theurapeutic management of hepatic trauma. A retrospective study comparing 2 series of cases in different (1997-1984 vs 2001-2008). Cir Esp 2011;89:439–47.

9. Kozar RA, Moore FA, Cothren CC, et al. Risk factors for hepatic morbidity following nonoperative management: multicenters study. Arch Surg 2006;141: 451–9.

10. Letoublon C, Chen Y, Arvieux C, et al. Delayed celiotomy or laparascopy as part of the nonoperative management of blunt hapatic trauma. World J Surg 2008;32: 1189–93.

11. Fang JF, Chen RJ, Wong YC, et al. Classification and treatment of pooling of contrast material on computed tomography scan of blunt hepatic trauma. J Trauma 2000;49: 1083–8.

12. Zargar M, Laal M. Liver trauma: operative and non-operative management. IJCRIMPH 2010;2(4):96–107.

13. Parks NA, Davis JW, Forman D, et al. Observation for nonoperative management of blunt liver injuries: how long is long enough? J Trauma 2011;70:626–9.

14. Pachter HL, Hofstetter SR. The current status of nonoperative management of adult blunt hepatic injuries. Am J Surg 1995;169:442–54.

15. Hoffer EK, Borsa JJ, Bloch RD, et al. Endovascular techniques in the damage control setting. Radiographics 1999;19:1340–8.

16. Tinkoff G, Esposito TJ, Reed J, et al. American association for the surgery of trauma organ injury scale 1: spleen, liver and kidney, validation based on the National Trauma Data Bank. J Am Coll Surg 2008;207:646–55.

17. Isenhour JL, Marx JA. Abdominal trauma. In: Marx JA, editor. Rosen's emergency medicine concepts and clinical practice. 7th edition. Philadelphia, PA: Elsevier; 2006. p. 414–34.

18. Brown CK, Dunn KA, Wilson K. Diagnostic evaluation of patients with blunt abdominal trauma: a decision analysis. Acad Emerg Med 2000;7:385–96.

19. Nishijima DK, Simel DL, Wisner DH, et al. Does this adult patient have a blunt intra-abdominal injury? JAMA 2012;307:1517–27.

20. Poletti PA, Mirvis SE, Shanmuganathan K, et al. Blunt abdominal truama patients: can organ injury be excluded without performing computed tomography? J Trauma 2004;57:1072–81.

21. Beck D, Marley R, Salvator A, et al. Prospective study of the clinical predictors of a positive abdominal computed tomography in blunt truama patients. J Trauma 2004;57:296–300.

22. Walter K. Radiographic evaluation of the patient with sport-related abdominal trauma. Curr Sports Med Rep 2007;6:115–9.

23. Shuman WP. CT of blunt abdominal truama in adults. Radiology 1997;205: 297–306.

24. Holmes JF, Wisner DH, McGahan JP, et al. Clinical prediction rules for identifying adults at very low risk for intra-abdominal injuries after blunt trauma. Ann Emerg Med 2009;54:575–84.

25. Deunk J, Brink M, Dekker HM, et al. Predictors for the selection of patients for abdominal CT after blunt abdominal truama: a proposal for a diagnostic algorithm. Ann Surg 2010;251:512–20.

26. Neal MD, Peitzman AB, Forsythe RM, et al. Over reliance on computed tomography imaging in patients with severe abdominal injury: is the delay worth the risk? J Trauma 2011;70:278–84.

27. Hoffman R, Nerlich M, Muggia-Sullam M, et al. Blunt abdominal trauma in cases of multiple trauma evaluated by ultrasonography: a prospective analysis of 291 patients. J Trauma 1992;32:452–8.

28. Cha JY, Kashuk JL, Sarin EL, et al. Diagnostic peritoneal lavage remains a valuable adjunct to modern imaging techniques. J Trauma 2009;67:330–6.

29. Peitzman AB, Richardson JD. Surgical treatment of injuries to the solid abdominal organs: a 50-year perspective from the Journal of Trauma. J Trauma 2010;69: 1011–21.

30. Pachter HL, Knudson MM, Esrig B, et al. Status of nonoperative management of blunt hepatic injuries in 1995: a multicenter experience with 404 patients. J Trauma 1996;40:31–8.

31. Asensio JA, Demetriades D, Chahwan S, et al. Approach to the management of complex hepatic injuries. J Trauma 2000;48:66–9.

32. Asensio JA, Roldan G, Petrone P, et al. Operative management and outcomes in 103 AAST-OIS grades IV and V complex hepatic injuries: trauma surgeons still need to operate, but angioembolization helps. J Trauma 2003;54:647–54.

33. Polanco P, Leon S, Pineda J, et al. Hepatic resection in the management of complex injury to the liver. J Trauma 2008;65:1264–70.

34. Richardson JD. Changes in the management of injuries to the liver and spleen. J Am Coll Surg 2005;200:648–69.

Blunt Bladder Injury

Ivette Guttmann, MD, Hamish A. Kerr, MD, MSc*

KEYWORDS

- Bladder rupture • Bladder contusion • Hematuria

KEY POINTS

- Bladder injury should be suspected when trauma is followed by gross hematuria, suprapubic or abdominal pain, and difficulty in voiding or the inability to void.
- Bladder rupture with blunt abdominal trauma is uncommon; however, because of its high mortality rate, recognition of the early signs and symptoms can be life saving.
- The most common type of injury is a bladder contusion, which is a diagnosis of exclusion.
- Extraperitoneal bladder ruptures are almost exclusively associated with a pelvic fracture.

INTRODUCTION

The abdomen has a large surface area with an absence of bony support. Protective equipment in this area could undermine athletic performance, making this area prone to potentially serious injury.[1] Fortunately, the bladder is located deep within the protective bony structures of the pelvis, making it fairly well protected from blunt sports-related trauma.

The bladder is a hollow organ that collects urine from the kidney. When the bladder is empty, it is protected, although not exempt, from injury behind the pelvic rami. An appropriate mechanism and sufficient force can still result in injury if a pelvic fracture is incurred. In the child, the pelvic bones are not fully developed, making the bladder more easily injured than in the adult.[2]

As the bladder fills, it rises just slightly above the pelvic structures, exposing itself to the unprotected abdomen and making it more vulnerable to blunt injury. In infants and young children, the urinary bladder is in the abdomen even when empty. The bladder usually descends into the pelvis by age 20 years.

EPIDEMIOLOGY

Sports-related trauma causes about 10% of all abdominal injury.[1] Bladder injuries occur in 1.6% of all blunt abdominal trauma cases.[2] Bladder rupture is uncommon

Disclosures: None.
Conflict of Interest: None.
Primary Care Sports Medicine Fellowship, Division of Internal Medicine and Pediatrics, Albany Medical College, 724 Watervliet-Shaker Road, Latham, NY 12110, USA
* Corresponding author.
E-mail address: kerrh@mail.amc.edu

Clin Sports Med 32 (2013) 239–246
http://dx.doi.org/10.1016/j.csm.2012.12.006
0278-5919/13/$ – see front matter

with blunt trauma because of its position; however, it has a mortality rate of 22% after blunt abdominal trauma.[3]

MECHANISM: MACROTRAUMATIC

Bladder injuries can be caused by high-energy blunt trauma that disrupts the bony pelvis such as a direct blow to a distended bladder or a penetrating injury. Of all bladder injuries, 60% to 85% are from blunt trauma and 15% to 40% are from a penetrating injury.[4] The most common non–sports-related mechanism of injury to the bladder is a motor vehicle collision. However, given the propensity of some sports for high-velocity contact and collision, injury to the bladder can occur. Overall, the most common sport to cause abdominal injury is cycling. Martial arts, softball, snowboarding, football, rugby, gymnastics, and hockey are just some of the sports with the capability to cause significant abdominal and subsequent bladder injury as a result of mechanisms such as acceleration, deceleration, and spearing. An example of such a force is a direct kick or blow to the abdomen during martial arts, a known discipline for having the potential to produce traumatic bladder injuries.[1] Gymnasts are not immune from this type of injury; for example, gymnasts may develop severe bruising around the lower abdomen and anterior superior iliac spine by performing the "beat maneuver" on the uneven bars. Gymnasts at the lower competitive levels typically perform this skill, which involves hanging from the high bar and dropping the anterior pelvis and hips onto the low bar, and are consequently are at risk for developing a bladder contusion.[5]

MECHANISM: MICROTRAUMATIC

Another sport that can also injure the bladder by causing repetitive jolting is long distance running, generating transient bladder contusions. This can be caused by a combination of exertional forces and intra-abdominal pressure producing repeated impact of the flaccid wall of the bladder against the bladder base. The bladder may be empty or nearly empty while the runner is in action. This permits apposition of the surfaces of the bladder. This is manifested as transient hematuria. The variability of the state of filling one's bladder from one occasion to another may therefore account for the inconsistency of occurrence of hematuria in the same runner.[6] It is thought that partial filling of the bladder will prevent this type of insult. The partially filled bladder will provide enough tautness to its walls to counteract such exertional forces and increased intra-abdominal pressure.

PATHOPHYSIOLOGY AND CLASSIFICATION

Bladder injuries are principally defined as contusions or bladder ruptures. Bladder rupture in the setting of blunt trauma may be classified as either extraperitoneal (70%–90% of cases) with leakage of urine limited to the perivesical space, or intraperitoneal (15%–25%), in which the peritoneal surface has been disrupted with concomitant urinary extravasation (**Fig. 1**), or it can be combined with both intraperitoneal and extraperitoneal rupture (5%–12%). Combined intraperitoneal and extraperitoneal bladder ruptures are mainly diagnosed during surgery.[7]

BLADDER CONTUSION

The most common type of bladder injury is a contusion. Bladder contusions, or a "bruised bladder," are relatively benign, and this is usually a diagnosis of exclusion. Bladder contusion is an incomplete or partial-thickness tear of the bladder mucosa or

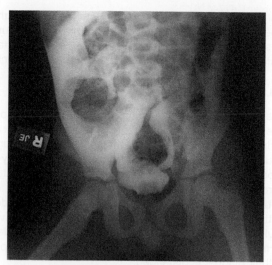

Fig. 1. Pediatric bladder trauma. Contrast material is visualized in the peritoneum in this child's abdomen during a cystogram. (*Courtesy of* Dr B. Dangman.)

muscularis, without complete loss of wall continuity. A segment of the bladder wall is bruised or contused, resulting in localized injury and hematoma.[2]

EXTRAPERITONEAL BLADDER RUPTURE

Extraperitoneal bladder rupture is commonly associated with a pelvic fracture (**Fig. 2**), and an intraperitoneal bladder rupture is usually a result of blunt lower abdominal force on a full bladder.

Most bladder injuries are related to blunt trauma on a distended bladder. The risk of bladder rupture increases with bladder distention. Perforation of an empty bladder is generally associated with a penetrating injury, either extrinsic or a bone fragment. Bladder ruptures are rare. Eighty-three percent of patients with bladder ruptures have pelvic fractures, but less than 10% of patients with pelvic fractures have bladder ruptures.[7] The protective effect of the pelvic ring is lost with a fracture of the anterior pubic arch, and these ruptures may occur from a direct laceration of the bladder by the

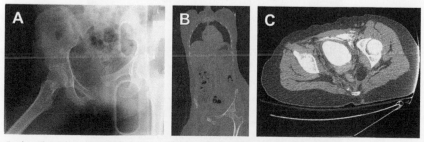

Fig. 2. (*A–C*) Radiograph showing pelvic rami and pubic symphysis disruption. (*B*) CT scan of abdomen and pelvis showing pelvic disruption plus left ileum fracture. (*C*) Cystogram showing extraperitoneal bladder rupture with contrast adjacent to the bladder. (*Courtesy of* Dr B. Dangman.)

bony fragments of the osseous pelvis. The anterolateral aspect of the bladder is the portion typically perforated by bony spicules. During this type of injury, the displaced pelvic bones transmit the force vector to the bladder, shearing the extraperitoneal bladder on the anterior lateral wall near its base and its fascial attachments.[8]

INTRAPERITONEAL BLADDER RUPTURE

The high incidence of intraperitoneal bladder rupture in patients without pelvic fracture favors the hypothesis that it results from a blow to the abdomen that compresses and ruptures a distended urinary bladder.[9] Intraperitoneal bladder rupture (**Fig. 3**) occurs when there is a sudden increase in intravesical pressure secondary to a blow to the pelvis or lower abdomen. This increased pressure results in a rupture of the dome, the weakest and most mobile part of the bladder.[7]

Intraperitoneal bladder rupture thus seems to be related to the degree of bladder distention at the time of injury, as well as to the magnitude of pelvic injury. Hence, a marathoner would not be susceptible to the same degree of bladder injury as would a downhill skier. However, all athletes can have bladder injuries, especially if they are competing while their bladder is distended.

CLINICAL PRESENTATION

Clinical signs of bladder injury are relatively nonspecific; however, a triad of symptoms is often present: gross hematuria, suprapubic or abdominal pain or tenderness, and difficulty in voiding or inability to void. Athletes will usually present with a history of trauma. They can pass small blood clots and often report dysuria and hematuria. However, athletes may also present with gross hematuria simply after participation in extreme physical activity such as long distance running.

Hematuria invariably accompanies all bladder injuries, but it may be transient or even microscopic. Because the bladder is a highly vascular organ, gross hematuria is the hallmark of a bladder rupture. Although grossly clear urine in a trauma patient

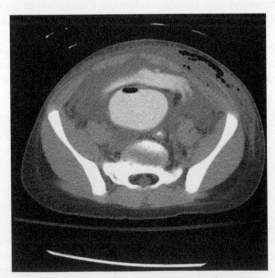

Fig. 3. Intraperitoneal bladder rupture showing contrast in the peritoneal cavity. (*Courtesy of* Dr B. Dangman.)

without a pelvic fracture virtually eliminates the possibility of a bladder rupture, more than 95% of bladder ruptures are associated with gross hematuria and fewer than 5% are associated with microscopic hematuria.[10] A normal urinalysis does not rule out bladder injury, and there should always be a high index of suspicion if the history and physical examination point to a probable intra-abdominal injury.

Exactly how much blood in the urine necessitates investigation is a point of controversy in the literature. In their series, Morgan and colleagues[11] reported that no ruptures were seen in patients with fewer than 25 red blood cells per high-power field, thus suggesting cystography is not needed in these cases of microhematuria. However, in pediatric patients, according to Abou-Jaoude and colleagues,[12] a threshold for radiological evaluation of greater than or equal to 20 red blood cells per high-power field would miss 25% of cases with bladder injury. They suggested that lower urogenital tract evaluation in pediatric trauma patients, especially in the presence of pelvic fractures, should be based as much on clinical judgment as on the presence of hematuria.

Bladder contusions can have transient hematuria or may even be clinically silent; however, the amount of hematuria does not indicate the degree of bladder injury. Nor does the ability to urinate exclude bladder injury or perforation. Bladder contusions are much more frequent and, as mentioned earlier, can present with no clinical signs, thereby making their incidence truly unknown because they can go undiagnosed.

Muscular contusions may be difficult to distinguish from visceral injury and may even coexist. Tenderness is usually only over the site of the contusion and worsens with contraction (Carnett sign) but improves after the muscle remains tense. Muscular contusions do not cause referred pain, but bladder injury will.[1]

Although bladder ruptures are rare in the athlete, a delay in diagnosis can increase their mortality. A bladder rupture is more clinically discernible than a bladder contusion, but a good history and physical examination that detail the sport in which the athlete was participating and how the injury occurred (mechanism of injury), as well as an evaluation of whether the athlete could have sustained a pelvic fracture, are essential for an accurate and timely diagnosis.

It is thus important to understand the mechanism of how an injury has been sustained and the anatomy of the abdomen. It is equally important to identify the signs associated with intraperitoneal, retroperitoneal, and pelvic trauma; to apply diagnostic and therapeutic procedures specific to abdominal trauma; and to understand the limitations and advantages of available diagnostic procedures. The immediate assessment of the athlete with abdominal injury must take into account the potential for the evolution of critical injuries.[13]

With bladder ruptures, an abdominal examination may reveal signs of peritoneal irritation, which include distention, guarding, and rebound tenderness. Absent bowel sounds and signs of peritoneal irritation indicate a possible intraperitoneal bladder rupture. A rectal examination should be performed to exclude rectal injury and, in men, to evaluate prostate position. If the prostate is "high riding" or elevated, it may further suggest proximal urethra and bladder disruption.[10] Unexplained abnormal serum electrolyte, blood urea nitrogen, and creatine levels should raise suspicion of an intraperitoneal rupture.[2]

DIAGNOSTIC EVALUATION

Diagnostic evaluation should include serial vital signs; this is the best method to suspect a diagnosis of an intra-abdominal injury. Diagnostic imaging is the most important tool in the assessment of the athlete with intra-abdominal injury. A static or computed tomography (CT) cystogram should be performed and can be used to diagnose bladder injury. The urinary bladder is a low-pressure and large-compliance storage system; intravesical pressure should be increased by bladder distention, or the injury may be easily missed. Cystography should be performed by filling the bladder with dilute contrast via a Foley catheter with at least 300 mL or until extravasation occurs. Incomplete distention of the bladder is related to failure of diagnosis. Postdrainage radiographs are essential to avoid missing 10% to 15% of injuries that are not seen initially.[2]

The usual indications for cystography, whether plain film or CT; are gross hematuria or the combination of a pelvic fracture and microscopic hematuria. The standard radiographic evaluation of all patients with blunt trauma includes an anteroposterior pelvic radiograph. If a pelvic fracture is visualized on the initial pelvic radiograph or suspected on physical examination, further imaging by CT of the abdomen and pelvis and inlet and outlet radiographs of the pelvis should be performed.[14] CT is clearly the method of choice for the evaluation of patients with blunt or penetrating abdominal and/or pelvic trauma. However, routine CT is not reliable in the diagnosis of bladder rupture. CT demonstrates intraperitoneal and extraperitoneal fluid but cannot differentiate urine from ascites.[13]

However, according to a study by Deck and colleagues[14] CT cystography is advocated over plain film cystography only for patients undergoing CT scanning for other injuries. Although it has its advantages of rapid assessment and the ability to detect small amounts of intraperitoneal or extraperitoneal fluid, it also has its disadvantages in terms of radiation exposure and cost. Furthermore, CT can have decreased interpretation resulting from bony fragments of a pelvic fracture.[14] However, with the advancement of CT technology, it has evolved to become the standard of care. Therefore, for gross hematuria, a CT scan of the abdomen and pelvis to evaluate the kidneys and a CT cystogram should be obtained (**Fig. 4**).

The diagnosis of bladder contusion is usually established by exclusion, and management usually includes observation alone, ensuring that hematuria resolves. However, some cases require catheter drainage. In a contused bladder, extravasation

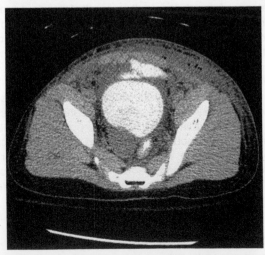

Fig. 4. CT cystogram indicating bladder rupture with contrast adjacent to the bladder. (*Courtesy of* Dr B. Dangman.)

is not apparent on cystography, but the bladder outline may be distorted. Its true incidence is hard to estimate because many contusions either are clinically silent and remain undiagnosed or are manifested by transient hematuria with negative cystography and receive no treatment.

Patients with large pelvic hematomas or bladder neck distortion may require catheter drainage until ambulatory or until there is sufficient restoration of normal anatomy with hematoma absorption, when prophylactic antibiotic therapy may be initiated.[2]

A child's bladder is primarily an intra-abdominal organ; therefore, blunt abdominal trauma in children typically results in intraperitoneal bladder injuries. An intraperitoneal rupture is more common in children because of this relative intra-abdominal position of the bladder and, thus, increased vulnerability to trauma.[10]

Intraperitoneal bladder ruptures, however, are far from being exclusive to children. An intraperitoneal rupture can occur as a result of an athlete sustaining a blunt trauma to the lower abdomen, and it is strongly associated with the presence of intraperitoneal free fluid. It is even more common with a full bladder.[15] An intraperitoneal rupture should always be managed by surgical exploration and repair if needed. This type of injury involves a high degree of force and, because of the severity of associated injuries, carries a high mortality rate.

Extraperitoneal bladder ruptures usually involve the anterolateral bladder surface near the bladder neck.[16] Extravasated contrast media infiltrates the extraperitoneal tissues. Extraperitoneal bladder ruptures occur mainly in athletes who have also sustained a pelvic fracture. Most isolated uncomplicated injuries can be managed with catheter drainage alone. A cystogram should be repeated on the 10th day; more than 85% of bladders will be healed by then. Prophylactic antibiotics are given while the catheter is in place. Most injuries treated in this manner are healed within 3 weeks of catheter drainage.[2]

Problems arise almost universally when diagnosis is delayed. Thus, transient or gross hematuria or lower abdominal pain or complaints of voiding, especially after an athletic injury or competition, requires further investigation.

PREVENTION

Despite the knowledge of injury patterns, effecting change remains extremely difficult, particularly in sports such as skiing, in which participants are frequently young "risk takers."[13] Prevention would be key, and the use of padding to prevent injury ideal. However, in most contact sports that would put an athlete at risk for blunt abdominal injury, padding would be impractical and even detrimental to performance. Therefore, it is important to remember to wear adequate protective equipment when possible and to keep the bladder empty during exercise or any competitive event.

ACKNOWLEDGMENTS

The images of pelvic fractures and bladder ruptures are all courtesy of Barbara Dangman, MD, Division of Pediatric Radiology, Department of Pediatrics, Children's Hospital at Albany Medical Center, Albany, NY. Dr Dangman's assistance in preparing this article is greatly appreciated.

REFERENCES

1. Brown DL. Genitourinary problems in the athlete. In: Birrer RB, O'Connor FG, editors. Sports Medicine for the Primary Care Physician. 3rd edition. Boca Raton, Florida: CRC Press; 2004. p. 751–60.

2. Gomez RG, Ceballos L, Coburn M, et al. Consensus statement on bladder injuries. BJU Int 2004;94(1):27–32.
3. Iverson AJ, Morey AF. Radiographic evaluation of suspected bladder rupture following blunt trauma: critical review. World J Surg 2001;25(12):1588–91.
4. Cass AS, Luxenberg M. Features of 164 bladder ruptures. J Urol 1987;138(4): 743–5.
5. Johnson M. Genitourinary. In: O'Connor, Francis G, editors. Sports medicine: just the facts. Columbus OH: McGraw-Hill; 2005. p. 157–61.
6. Blacklock NJ. Bladder trauma in the long-distance runner. Am J Sports Med 1979;7(4):239–41.
7. Zacharias C, Robinson JD, Linnau KF, et al. Blunt urinary bladder trauma. Curr Probl Diagn Radiol 2012;41(4):140–1.
8. McCort J. Bladder injury and pelvic fractures. Emerg Radiol 1994;1(1):47–51.
9. Peters P. Genitourinary trauma. In: Walsh P, Retik A, Vaughan E, editors. Campbell's urology. 6th edition. St Louis (MO): Saunders; 1992. p. 2571–93.
10. Brandes S, Borrelli J Jr. Pelvic fracture and associated urologic injuries. World J Surg 2001;25(12):1578–87.
11. Morgan DE, Nallamala LK, Kenney PJ, et al. CT cystography: radiographic and clinical predictors of bladder rupture. AJR Am J Roentgenol 2000;174(1):89–95.
12. Abou-Jaoude WA, Sugarman JM, Fallat ME, et al. Indicators of genitourinary tract injury or anomaly in cases of pediatric blunt trauma. J Pediatr Surg 1996;31(1): 86–9 [discussion: 90].
13. Ryan JM. Abdominal injuries and sport. Br J Sports Med 1999;33(3):155–60.
14. Deck AJ, Shaves S, Talner L, et al. Current experience with computed tomographic cystography and blunt trauma. World J Surg 2001;25(12):1592–6.
15. Shin SS, Jeong YY, Chung TW, et al. The sentinel clot sign: a useful CT finding for the evaluation of intraperitoneal bladder rupture following blunt trauma. Korean J Radiol 2007;8(6):492–7.
16. Sandler CM, Hall JT, Rodriguez MB, et al. Bladder injury in blunt pelvic trauma. Radiology 1986;158(3):633–8.

Male Genital Trauma in Sports

Stanley R. Hunter, MD[a], Timothy S. Lishnak, MD, CAQSM[b],
Andria M. Powers, MD[c], David K. Lisle, MD, CAQSM[b,d],*

KEYWORDS

- Testicular hemotoma • Rupture • Urethral injury • Urethrogram
- Scrotal hematocele

KEY POINTS

- If testicular hematoma or rupture is suspected on examination, evaluate with Doppler ultrasound. Positive ultrasound evaluation or ambiguous ultrasound evaluation requires early surgical exploration.
- If urethral injury is suspected on examination, a retrograde urethrogram must be performed before the placement of a Foley catheter. If the urethrogram is positive, urologic surgery consult is required.
- If penile injury is suspected on examination, urologic surgery consult is required.
- Surgery is the definitive diagnostic and treatment for testicular rupture, severe scrotal hematocele, severe intratesticular hematoma, testicular avulsion, testicular torsion, urethral disruption, and penile cavernosal injury. Early surgical intervention improves outcomes in testicular rupture, severe scrotal hematocele, severe intratesticular hematoma, and testicular torsion, and does no harm in other injuries. A low threshold for early surgical consult is prudent.

BACKGROUND AND MECHANISMS

Male genital trauma is a rare but potentially serious sports injury. Although such an injury can occur by many different mechanisms, including falls, collisions, straddle injuries, kicks, and equipment malfunction, the clinical presentation is typically homogeneous, characterized by pain and swelling. Almost all sports-related male genital

Funding Sources: Nil.
Conflicts of Interest: Nil.
[a] Milton Family Practice, Department of Family Medicine, University of Vermont College of Medicine, 111 Colchester Avenue, Burlington, VT 05401, USA; [b] Department of Family Medicine, University of Vermont College of Medicine, 235 Rowell, 106 Carrigan Drive, Burlington, VT 05405, USA; [c] Department of Radiology, University of Vermont College of Medicine, 111 Colchester Avenue, Burlington, VT 05401, USA; [d] Division of Sports Medicine, Department of Orthopaedics and Rehabilitation, University of Vermont College of Medicine, 192 Tilley Drive, South Burlington, VT 05403-7205, USA
* Corresponding author. Division of Sports Medicine, Department of Orthopaedics and Rehabilitation, 192 Tilley Drive, South Burlington, VT 05403-7205.
E-mail address: David.Lisle@vtmednet.org

injury comes from blunt force trauma, with involvement of scrotal structures far more common than penile structures.[1] Most injuries can be treated conservatively, but catastrophic testicular injury must first be ruled out. Despite being relatively uncommon compared with other sports injuries, more than half of all testicular injuries are sustained during sports.[1] Ninety percent of blunt testicular injuries are isolated; 5% are associated with penile injury, and less than 2% are bilateral.[2]

BLUNT TRAUMA WITH SUSPECTED TESTICULAR RUPTURE

Testicular rupture is characterized by rupture of the tunica albuginea and extravasation of seminiferous tubules.[1] Severity may vary from a small laceration with minimal extravasation to complete parenchymal destruction.[3] The mechanism is usually via a direct blow with compression of the scrotum against the pelvis or thigh.[3] According to a 1946 case report, approximately 50 kg compression is required to cause rupture, although this number is not substantiated or referenced.[4] This force is likely less in the setting of tumor or other structural compromise, leading to the possibility of uncovering an underlying condition from trauma.[3]

Testicular mobility, the cremasteric reflex, and the strength of the tunica albuginea all contribute to making testicular rupture uncommon.[2] Most male genital injuries from sports are minor contusions that resolve without treatment.[1]

Clinical History

Presenting symptoms include severe pain, nausea, emesis, and sometimes syncope.[3] Usually the time and mechanism of trauma are obvious. When a patient presents late, a history of improvement of symptoms does not rule out rupture. Pain will improve gradually, even with untreated testicular rupture.[3]

Physical Examination and Testing

The goal of the physical examination and adjunctive testing is to separate those injuries requiring surgical exploration from those that may be treated conservatively. An examination may be difficult due to the presence of pain and swelling, but the location of swelling can have prognostic value. One set of authors describes an examination technique of grasping the neck of the scrotum with 3 fingers posterosuperiorly to the involved testis and the thumb anteriorly. Swelling below the thumb implicates testicular injury, epididymal injury, or hydrocele. Swelling above thumb implicates incarcerated hernia or spermatic cord injury.[5]

Swelling, ecchymosis, and tenderness to palpation are typically appreciated on examination.[1] A hemiscrotal hematocele is often apparent as a tender mass larger than a baseball and causing loss of rugae of the scrotal skin. Such a hematocele is common in association with testicular rupture and will not transilluminate.[3]

Imaging

Adjunctive imaging is valuable due to poor specificity of examination findings and the necessity for a low threshold for surgical exploration in suspected testicular injury. An ultrasound scan of 7.5 to 10 MHz with a linear array transducer became a standard in the evaluation of testicular trauma in the mid 1980s.[2,6] Doppler ultrasound studies can evaluate perfusion of a jeopardized testicle.[7] Although several studies report discordant results about the utility of ultrasound in diagnosing intrascrotal injuries, some of the discrepancy seems to be due to changes and improvements in ultrasound technology in the last 25 years. One 2008 French study performed retrospectively on a series of patients compiled sensitivity and specificity estimates for ultrasound of various types of intrascrotal injury.[8] All patients in this study underwent both ultrasound and the diagnostic gold standard of surgical exploration (Table 1).

Ultrasound was found highly sensitive for detecting testicular rupture and avulsion, but relatively poor at detecting epididymal injury. Although sensitivity was low for epididymal injury, the authors report that epididymal injury was always accompanied by severe testicular injury that was easily detected and, overall, ultrasound tended not to underestimate injury (Figs. 1–4).[8] Highest accuracy is obtained in ultrasound evaluation by looking for signs consistent with the loss of testicular contour definition, heterogeneity of the testicular parenchyma, or breach of the tunica albuginea. Looking exclusively for breach of the tunica albuginea results in lower sensitivity.[8]

Differential

The history may suggest an obvious traumatic event and mechanism, although nontraumatic causes must be considered. In cases not involving trauma or collision, the differential for scrotal injuries includes epididymitis, orchitis, incarcerated inguinal hernia, testicular torsion, appendicular torsion, hydrocele, hematocele, and neoplasm.[3,5] Clothing and gear also deserve consideration. One case study reported a spermatic cord hematoma caused by poorly fitting protective football equipment and a hip spica used to treat a previous injury.[5]

Testicular torsion

Four percent to 8% of cases of testicular torsion result from trauma, and torsion should be in the differential for delayed presentation of pain after scrotal trauma.[9]

History Testicular torsion usually presents with diffuse, unilateral pain and tenderness. Half of the patients may have nausea and vomiting and 25% will have fever. Urinary symptoms or discharge are not characteristic. Torsion of the appendix testis presents similarly. Acute pain and swelling in a testicle without recent trauma should be treated as torsion unless proven otherwise.[9]

Examination signs The 2 best clinical signs supporting testicular torsion are absent cremasteric reflex and high and horizontal testicular lie. The literature is divided on the importance of the lack of a cremasteric reflex with some authors reporting the absence to be 99% sensitive[9] and others reporting the absence of a cremasteric reflex as an unreliable finding.[10] Although a high transverse lie is a useful clinical finding, lie can also be vertical and/or low, and no examination finding can rule out torsion.[10]

Blue dot sign, a small area of cyanosis on the scrotal skin, is best seen with the skin stretched, either with or without transillumination, and indicates torsion of the appendix testis.

Table 1
Accuracy of ultrasonography for blunt scrotal trauma

Injury Type	Sensitivity	Specificity	PPV	NPV
Testicular rupture	100%	65%	73%	100%
Hematocele	87%	89%	95%	72%
Testicular hematoma	71%	79%	45%	91%
Testicular avulsion	100%	97%	50%	100%
Epididymal injury	57%	85%	50%	88%

Data from Guichard G, El Ammari J, Del Coro C, et al. Accuracy of ultrasonography in diagnosis of testicular rupture after blunt scrotal trauma. Urology 2008;71(1):52–6.

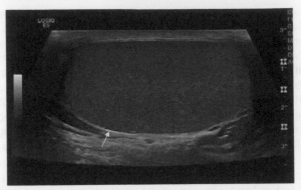

Fig. 1. Sagittal image of a normal testicle. The testis is homogeneous in echotexture with uniform mid level echoes. A thin, well-defined hyperechoic rim surrounding the testis represents the capsule, composed of tunica albuginea (*arrow*).

Prehn sign, the relief of discomfort with lifting of the testicle on the affected side, indicates epididymoorchitis but is not clinically useful due to low sensitivity and specificity.

Imaging The most important modality for diagnosing torsion is ultrasound, and a snail-shaped spermatic cord mass is characteristic.[10] Doppler ultrasound may show compromise of blood flow to the testicle.

Treatment Definitive treatment of torsion is surgical, with detorsion, orchiopexy, and exploration of the contralateral side. Within 6 hours, rates of salvage are greater than 90%. At 12 hours, salvage drops to 50%, and at 24 hours salvage is only 10%. Beyond 24 hours, salvage is minimal.[9] Before surgery, manual detorsion may be attempted. Start by turning the involved testis laterally, because two-thirds of torsions involve medial rotation. If symptoms and tactile feel indicate, the physician may secondarily attempt medial rotation. Manual detorsion is successful in 26% to 80% of patients, and success can be inferred by a reduction in pain.[9] Surgical orchiopexy is still indicated to prevent recurrence.

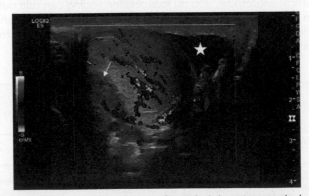

Fig. 2. Sagittal image of testis after a low-grade groin injury. Intratesticular hematoma. A hypoechoic, ovoid region with decreased to absent blood flow in the testis represents intratesticular hematoma (*arrow*). The overall contour of the testis is preserved and the capsule is intact. Anechoic fluid around the testis represents a hydrocele (*star*).

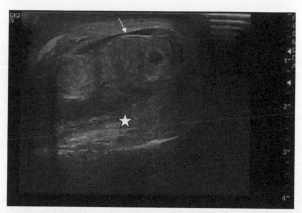

Fig. 3. Sagittal image of the testis after direct trauma with a baseball. Testicular rupture. The testis is heterogeneous with lobulated, abnormal morphology; there is little to no normal-appearing testicular tissue. The hyperechoic capsule (*arrow*) is discontinuous and poorly seen. Surrounding echogenic material reflects hematoma (*star*).

Hematocele

Hematocele is hemorrhage into the tunica vaginalis and commonly accompanies testicular rupture. Hematoceles do not transilluminate, and because of an association with testicular rupture, traumatic hematoceles require ultrasound evaluation of the testicles. Clinically, hematoceles often make examination difficult by causing swelling, making palpation of deeper structures difficult, and contributing to tenderness.

Even an isolated hematocele may require surgical drainage because a tense hematocele can cause testicular atrophy by pressure.[2] An undrained hematocele can also cause delayed testicular loss because of secondary infection, irrespective of antibiosis.[11] Untreated most hematoceles resorb in 1 to 2 months, during which time walking, driving, and leg crossing can be painful.[11]

Hydrocele

Hydrocele is an accumulation of serous fluid within the tunica vaginalis. It does transilluminate.

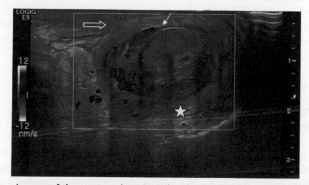

Fig. 4. Transverse image of the ruptured testis with color Doppler imaging. The central tissue is devascularized. A rim of vascular tissue represents a portion of viable testis, although it is abnormally heterogeneous and discontinuous from the rest of the organ. The testicular capsule is discontinuous (*arrow*). Echogenic, heterogeneous material surrounding the testis represents hematoma (*star*). The overlying scrotal skin is thickened and edematous (*open arrow*).

Treatment

General

A low threshold for surgical exploration must be maintained given the high rate of salvageability with early operation. Surgical exploration is reasonable if pain or swelling limits the ability to perform a good examination and ultrasound evaluation.

Conservative

Conservative treatment consists of bed rest, ice, elevation of bilateral lower extremities and scrotum, and nonsteroidal anti-inflammatory drug therapy. An athletic supporter or compression shorts may be useful for scrotal support. Use of a wheelchair can improve comfort if ambulation is painful.[5]

Surgical

With moderate or high suspicion for testicular rupture, torsion, epididymal injury, contusion with hematocele, or other internal structural defect, surgery should not be delayed. Multiple studies have shown better outcomes with early surgical intervention, generally defined as within 72 hours of injury.[2,11,12] A seminal article from 1969 reported an 80% rate of salvage in testicular rupture with operation within 3 days of injury, but only 33% salvage for operation between days 4 and 9, and 30% salvage for operations from 10 to 36 days.[12] Although less severe, contusion with hematocele also requires surgical intervention. A 1988 study reported that delayed surgery was required in 40% of cases of contusion with hematocele with a 15% rate of orchiectomy at surgery. Early surgery in that series resulted in a 0% rate of orchiectomy among 19 patients. The cause of most delayed losses was infection or unresorbed hematoma, even though all conservatively managed patients received prophylactic antibiotics.[11] A 1991 series of 91 incidents of testicular trauma, 72 of which were blunt, reported 21% testicular loss with early conservative management versus 6% loss with early surgery.[2] Furthermore, some authors report that even in the absence of testicular rupture, evacuation of a hematocele may reduce inflammation, pressure, and risk of atrophy.[12]

RETURN TO PLAY AND RESTRICTIONS

Return to play without limitation is allowed when injury symptoms and surgical and traumatic wounds have resolved.[9] Pain usually decreases proportionally to reduction in swelling.[5]

The American Academy of Pediatrics supports unrestricted sports participation for children with a single testicle or an undescended testicle but recommends consideration of protective equipment in sports with high relative risk of injury.[13]

PROTECTIVE EQUIPMENT AND SPORTS-SPECIFIC GUIDELINES

The National Operating Committee on Standards in Athletic Equipment, which regulates most protective athletic equipment, does not have standards for genitourinary equipment. No data exist to support use of an athletic cup, and design and manufacture are not regulated. Nonetheless, use of an athletic cup does make intuitive sense for some sports.[1] Common sense may be the best way to choose when an athletic cup is indicated, as no rating exists for the incidence of traumatic genital injury in sports.

Sports may be divided into noncontact, limited-contact, contact, and collision.[1,13] Collision sports, such as football, hockey, and rodeo, involve frequent and intentional high-energy impacts. Contact sports such as basketball involve frequent contact but with less energy.[13] Limited contact sports, such as baseball and bicycling, generally do not involve contact but may occasionally have high-energy contact. Clinician common sense comes into play because this categorization of sports does not separate out frequency of contact, energy of contact, or likelihood of genital involvement. Kidney injuries, for example, are at least as frequent from the limited-contact sports of bicycling and horseback riding as from the collision sport of football.[14] Some noncontact sports such as power lifting have moderate potential for injury, but are unlikely to involve genital trauma.

In making recommendations, the clinician should also remember that testicular injury is infrequent. A review of 4.4 million athlete exposures (defined as 1 athlete in 1 game or practice) from 1995 to 1997, found football to have a higher risk of testicular injury than baseball, basketball, soccer, or wrestling, but the incidence of testicular injury was universally low. Football had 9.2 testicular injuries per million athlete-exposures, ahead of soccer with 7.8, basketball with 2.3, wrestling with 1.9, and baseball with 0.[14] For comparison, football had 1080 head, neck, or spine injuries per million athlete-exposures, and that did not include mild traumatic brain injury, which had 594 incidents per million athlete-exposures.

In addition to a protective cup for high-risk sports, others recommend risk counseling and offering sperm banking for adults with only 1 viable testicle due to prior injury, nondescent, or cancer.[9] Some centers with andrology laboratories can perform sperm recovery after severe testicular trauma in monorchid patients using percutaneous epididymal sperm extraction or direct testicular sperm extraction from surgical specimens.[7]

PENILE TRAUMA

Acute penile trauma in sports is much less common even than scrotal trauma, probably because of the protected physical location, the relative invulnerability of the non-turgid penis to blunt injury, and the fact that blunt injury far exceeds penetrating injury as a mechanism in sports. The posterior urethra is the penile region most likely to sustain crush injury because of its immobility and proximity to the pelvis,[1] and the membranous urethra, which crosses the urogenital diaphram 2 to 3 cm posterior to the symphysis pubis, is the region most at risk in pelvic fracture.[1] Blunt penile injury suggests a high-energy collision, and 5% to 10% of urethral injuries are associated with pelvic fracture.[1] Anterior urethral injuries usually result from compression against the pubic symphysis.[1]

EXAMINATION

The most useful signs of urethral injury are blood at the meatus, perineal ecchymosis, hematocele, urinary retention, and high-riding prostate.[1] If urethral injury is suspected, retrograde urethrogram should be obtained before attempting Foley catheter placement. Both penile and urethral injuries require surgical exploration.[15]

REFERENCES

1. Styn NR, Wan J. Urologic sports injuries in children. Curr Urol Rep 2010;11(2): 114–21.
2. Cass AS, Luxenberg M. Testicular injuries. Urology 1991;37(6):528–30.
3. Wasko R, Goldstein AG. Traumatic rupture of the testicle. J Urol 1966;95(5): 721–3.
4. Wesson MB. Traumatism of the testicle; report of a case of traumatic rupture of a solitary testicle. Urol Cutaneous Rev 1946;50:16–9.

5. Bowman JR, Anton M. Spermatic cord hematoma in a collegiate football player: a case report. J Athl Train 1998;33(1):65–8.
6. Bhatt S, Dogra VS. Role of US in testicular and scrotal trauma. Radiographics 2008;28(6):1617–29.
7. Gadda F, Spinelli MG, Cozzi G, et al. Emergency testicular sperm extraction after scrotal trauma in a patient with a history of contralateral orchiopexy for cryptorchidism: case report and review of the literature. Fertil Steril 2012;97(5):1074–7.
8. Guichard G, El Ammari J, Del Coro C, et al. Accuracy of ultrasonography in diagnosis of testicular rupture after blunt scrotal trauma. Urology 2008;71(1):52–6.
9. Sandella B, Hartmann B, Berkson D, et al. Testicular conditions in athletes: torsion, tumors, and epididymitis. Curr Sports Med Rep 2012;11(2):92–5.
10. Mellick LB. Torsion of the testicle: it is time to stop tossing the dice. Pediatr Emerg Care 2012;28(1):80–6.
11. Cass AS, Luxenberg M. Value of early operation in blunt testicular contusion with hematocele. J Urol 1988;139(4):746–7.
12. Gross M. Rupture of the testicle: the importance of early surgical treatment. J Urol 1969;101(2):196–7.
13. Rice SG. American Academy of Pediatrics Council on Sports Medicine and Fitness. Medical conditions affecting sports participation. Pediatrics 2008; 121(4):841–8.
14. Grinsell MM, Butz K, Gurka MJ, et al. Sport-related kidney injury among high school athletes. Pediatrics 2012;130(1):e40–5.
15. Ferlise VJ, Haranto VH, Ankem MK, et al. Management of penetrating scrotal injury. Pediatr Emerg Care 2002;18(2):95–6.

Closed Lung Trauma

Jeffrey P. Feden, MD

KEYWORDS

- Thoracic trauma • Pneumothorax • Pneumomediastinum • Pulmonary contusion

KEY POINTS

- Blunt thoracic trauma can cause minor abrasions and contusions to the chest wall, rib fractures, and serious injury to the vital structures contained within the thoracic cage.
- Pneumothorax, hemothorax, pulmonary contusion, and pneumomediastinum are examples of pulmonary injuries that have been described after chest trauma during sports participation.
- The spectrum of clinical presentations ranges from subtle to potentially life threatening and may require emergency intervention.
- Chest radiographs and CT of the chest are the diagnostic studies of choice for blunt thoracic injury in the appropriate clinical setting.
- There are no specific guidelines for returning to sports after pulmonary injury, and available recommendations are based primarily on limited experience and case reports.

INTRODUCTION

The chest wall is composed of bony, cartilaginous, and muscular structures that serve to protect the thoracic organs and other vital structures, such as the trachea and great vessels. Blunt trauma to the chest wall may cause injury to these underlying structures, and clinical presentations can range from subtle to immediately life threatening (**Table 1**). Traumatic lung injury can occur from direct force, barotrauma, or rapid deceleration of the organs against the inner chest wall. Such injuries include pneumothorax, hemothorax, and pulmonary contusion. Pneumomediastinum may also result from bronchoalveolar disruption. Because of the potential complications of these conditions, athletes with thoracic trauma demand careful evaluation.

THE PRIMARY SURVEY

Initial assessment of athletes with thoracic trauma follows the standard principles of Advanced Trauma Life Support, with immediate attention to A: Airway with cervical spine immobilization, B: Breathing and ventilation, and C: Circulation with hemorrhage control.[1] The goal of this primary survey is to simultaneously identify and manage

Disclosures: None.
Department of Emergency Medicine, Alpert Medical School of Brown University, 593 Eddy Street, Claverick 2, Providence, RI 02903, USA
E-mail address: jfeden@lifespan.org

Table 1
Clinical signs and symptoms of pulmonary injury

Pneumothorax	Hemothorax	Pneumomediastinum	Pulmonary Contusion
Dyspnea	Dyspnea	Dyspnea	Dyspnea
Pleuritic chest pain	Chest pain	Retrosternal chest pain Neck pain Dysphonia Dysphagia Odynophagia Cough	Chest pain Hemoptysis
Tachypnea	Tachypnea	Subcutaneous emphysema	Tachypnea
Tachycardia	Tachycardia	Hamman crunch	Hypoxia
Anxiety	Anxiety	Fever	Wheezing
Hyperresonance to percussion	Dullness to percussion		Rales
Diminished breath sounds	Diminished breath sounds		
Tension PTX: Hypotension Hypoxia Tracheal deviation Distended neck veins	*Massive hemothorax:* Hypotension		

life-threatening injuries, such as airway obstruction, tension pneumothorax, massive hemothorax, open pneumothorax, flail chest with pulmonary contusion, and cardiac tamponade. Stabilization of the ABCs is mandatory before addressing less-threatening injuries and completing a more comprehensive evaluation. At the athletic venue, the decision to transport to an emergency department is based on the severity and mechanism of injury, in addition to the presence of respiratory compromise, hemodynamic instability, or clinical concern for potential decompensation.

PNEUMOTHORAX
Background

Pneumothorax (PTX) is defined simply as a collection of air within the pleural space. PTX can occur spontaneously or as a result of pleural injury with or without rib fracture after blunt trauma. Penetrating trauma, barotrauma, and iatrogenic causes of PTX are also well recognized. The negative intrathoracic pressure created during the inspiratory phase of respiration increases the tendency of air to leak into the pleural space, and air enters the pleural space until the pressure gradient is equalized.[2] Traumatic PTX can result from laceration of the visceral pleura by a fractured rib or from an abrupt increase in airway pressures and bronchial or alveolar rupture (eg, barotrauma). Traumatic PTX is a rare complication of athletic participation but has been reported in contact and collision sports, such as ice hockey,[3] football,[3,4] rugby,[5] and soccer.[6] Barotrauma related to scuba diving[7] and Valsalva maneuvers during weightlifting[8] can also produce PTX. Tension PTX can develop in the setting of a 1-way valve effect, whereby air accumulates in the pleural space with each breath but cannot escape (**Fig. 1**). Pressure in the affected hemithorax rises and produces tension. This leads to worsening hypoxia, mediastinal shift, decreased cardiac output, and death if left untreated.

The largest series of sports-related PTX was published by Kizer and MacQuarrie[9] and documents 20 cases over a 5-year period. All but 1 case were due to blunt chest trauma.

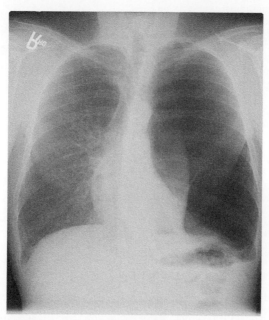

Fig. 1. Chest radiograph demonstrating left-sided tension PTX with resulting mediastinal shift to the right. (*Courtesy of* Robert Tubbs, MD, Providence, RI.)

Although 9 sports were involved, 11 cases were related to skiing or snowboarding. Other high-energy trauma, such as falls during equestrian sports, has also been associated with PTX.[10] Regardless of the mechanism, complications of PTX can be life threatening and must be considered in symptomatic athletes with chest trauma.

Diagnosis and Management

Diagnosis of PTX is commonly made by history and physical examination. Dyspnea with pleuritic chest pain is the classic presentation of PTX. Other clinical manifestations include tachypnea, tachycardia, anxiety, and hyperresonance to percussion and diminished lung sounds on the affected side. Late findings, or findings associated with tension pneumothorax, might include altered mental status, hypoxia, hypotension, distended neck veins, and tracheal deviation away from the affected side.[2] Infrequently, PTX may be asymptomatic.[11] Clinical suspicion for any thoracic injury should be further evaluated with chest radiographs. Conventional chest radiography (CXR) has long been the initial screening test after trauma. CXR is widely available, noninvasive, and inexpensive and offers a wealth of information. The supine anteroposterior CXR often used in trauma has poor sensitivity, however, and is unreliable in making the diagnosis.[2,12–14] With a small PTX, air accumulates in the anterobasal pleural space and may not be seen in the supine position.[13] The deep sulcus sign, an exaggerated lateral costovertebral angle (**Fig. 2**), may be the only clue.[15] Upright CXR in stable patients is the preferred technique, because it allows for better visualization of an apical air collection. If upright CXR is not possible, then bedside thoracic ultrasound has proved more sensitive than supine radiography for detection of PTX in blunt trauma patients.[12]

A growing body of literature supports multidetector CT for the diagnosis of thoracic injuries due to its superior sensitivity compared with CXR.[13] With the growth of CT use in trauma, the entity known as occult PTX has emerged. Occult PTX, by definition, is

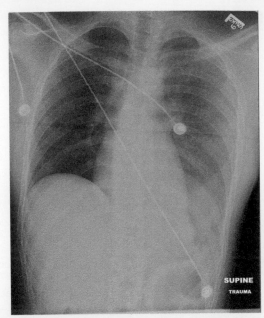

Fig. 2. Supine chest radiograph demonstrating a left-sided PTX and deep sulcus sign. This represents an abnormally deepened left costophrenic angle due to accumulation of air in the anterior and basal pleural space. (*Courtesy of* Robert Tubbs, MD, Providence, RI.)

identified only by CT scan and otherwise may go unrecognized.[14,16] Much of the existing data, however, are based on motor vehicle and other major trauma, and its clinical relevance to the athletic population remains unclear. Regardless, observation is a reasonably safe strategy in the management of traumatic occult PTX.[16,17]

Initial management of PTX focuses on an assessment of the airway, breathing, and circulation. Supplemental 100% oxygen should be administered immediately.[2] Respiratory distress and/or hemodynamic instability may be signs of tension PTX and must be addressed promptly because cardiovascular collapse and death can result. Treatment of tension PTX is accomplished by needle decompression, in which a 14G or 16G needle is inserted in the 2nd intercostal space in the midclavicular line to relieve pressure. Successful decompression is signaled by a rush of air and clinical improvement, and traditional placement of a large-bore chest tube to allow for lung re-expansion must follow.

Apart from tension pneumothorax, clinical management of PTX has evolved over the years and is based on the type and size of PTX in conjunction with the clinical presentation of the patient. The American College of Chest Physicians published consensus recommendations for the management of spontaneous PTX in 2001.[18] Clinically stable patients with a small PTX (<3 cm apex-to-cupola distance; the cupola is the superior pleural dome) may be managed with observation alone and discharged from the emergency department after 3 to 6 hours if repeat CXR excludes progression. A follow-up CXR should be obtained again in no more than 2 days to ensure resolution. Aspiration or tube thoracostomy is unnecessary except in cases where the PTX enlarges. A large PTX (>3 cm apex-to-cupola distance) in clinically stable patients should be re-expanded by insertion of a small-bore percutaneous catheter or large-bore (16F–22F) chest tube, and these patients are typically admitted to the hospital. Clinical stability is defined as respiratory rate less than 24 breaths/min, heart rate between 60 and 120 beats/min, normal blood pressure, room air oxygen saturation greater than 90%, and the ability to speak in whole sentences between breaths. Unstable patients with a large PTX should be hospitalized with a chest catheter, the size of which depends on clinical stability. In contrast to primary spontaneous PTX, secondary spontaneous PTX occurs in the setting of underlying lung disease. A more conservative approach is taken in these patients, with recommendations for hospital observation and a lower threshold for insertion of a chest catheter.

Similar consensus guidelines for the management of traumatic PTX are lacking, but treatment generally parallels that of spontaneous PTX. There is some evidence that stable patients with a simple traumatic PTX can be safely managed without chest drain insertion.[19] Otherwise, simple aspiration or chest tube thoracostomy is an effective strategy.[2] Obeid and colleagues[20] demonstrated the value of treating simple traumatic PTX with catheter aspiration in a small group of patients, although only 1 of these cases was due to blunt trauma. Other studies have similarly concluded that catheter aspiration is a successful, cost-effective alternative in patients with smaller pneumothoraces.[21,22] Tube thoracostomy is necessary for large pneumothoraces or for failure of aspiration. The chest tube is removed after the absence of an air leak with the tube to water seal is documented by CXR.[23]

Return to Play

There are no specific guidelines for returning to sports after traumatic pneumothorax. Timelines for return to play are based largely on case reports and expert opinion and range from 2 to 10 weeks.[4,11] Goal-oriented return to activity has been proposed rather than time-based return, consisting of progressive activity guided by symptoms.[4] Pain is most likely the limiting factor. Return to play should not be allowed before radiographic resolution of the PTX. Otherwise, available data suggest that return to play can occur at approximately 3 to 4 weeks after a traumatic PTX has resolved.[11] Treatment with a chest tube does not seem to affect these recommendations. Lastly, a flack jacket may be used for added chest wall protection.

Air Travel

With athletes and teams frequently traveling long distances by plane, the question of safe air travel after PTX occasionally arises. The primary concern over air travel relates to Boyle's law, which states that the absolute volume and pressure of a given mass of confined gas are inversely proportional. As altitude increases, barometric pressure decreases (although this is limited in a pressurized aircraft cabin). Theoretically, a volume of air trapped in the pleural cavity (PTX) expands and may convert a simple PTX into a tension PTX. The *Medical Guidelines for Airline Travel*[24] state that PTX is an absolute contraindication to air travel. Also, air travel should be safe by 2 to 3 weeks after successful drainage of a PTX.[24] A small prospective study by Cheatham and Safcsak[25] attempted to validate this recommendation. They found that 10 patients successfully completed air travel at least 14 days (mean 17.5 ± 4.9) after radiographic resolution of traumatic PTX without in-flight symptoms. One of 2 patients who flew before 2 weeks developed in-flight respiratory distress, suggesting recurrence. Therefore, they concluded that air travel at 2 weeks after radiographic resolution of a PTX is safe.

HEMOTHORAX
Background

Hemothorax, defined by a collection of blood within the pleural cavity, can result from aortic injury, myocardial rupture, or injuries to the hilum, intercostal vessels, or mammary vessels. In the setting of blunt trauma, PTX often accompanies hemorrhage and is termed, *hemopneumothorax*. Hemopneumothorax is more likely to result from high-energy blunt trauma or penetrating thoracic injury, but it may be caused by pulmonary laceration from rib fractures in minor trauma as well. There is only 1 sports-reported case of hemopneumothorax in the medical literature related to pulmonary trauma, occurring in a 34-year-old Japanese male club football player after being tackled.[26] This injury was associated with multiple rib fractures, pulmonary contusion, and a traumatic pulmonary pseudocyst. Hemothorax has been described rarely from blunt aortic rupture,[27] and aortic injury from posterior sternoclavicular joint dislocation also has the potential to produce hemothorax.[28]

Diagnosis and Management

Hemothorax is similar to PTX in that a collection of blood within the pleural space can reduce vital capacity, increase intrathoracic pressure, and compromise respiratory and cardiovascular function. Clinical presentation resembles that of pneumothorax, except that dullness to percussion may be evident on the affected side rather than hyperresonance. Hypotension can result from hemorrhagic shock. After assessment and stabilization of the airway, breathing, and circulation, the initial diagnostic study is an upright chest radiograph (CXR). Fluid collections greater than approximately 300 mL can be identified as fluid that blunts the costophrenic angle on upright CXR. As much as 1000 mL of blood may be missed on supine CXR because it produces only a mild diffuse hazy appearance.[29] CT scan has excellent sensitivity and complements CXR.

Bilello and colleagues[30] suggest that occult or small hemothorax (measured as <1.5-cm thickness of dependent fluid on CT) can be observed unless it increases in size. Guidelines published by the Eastern Association for the Surgery of Trauma recommend large-bore (36F–42F) tube thoracostomy as the initial treatment of choice for adequate drainage of all hemothoraces, regardless of size. Traditional indications for urgent thoracotomy for massive hemothorax or persistent hemorrhage include more than 1500 mL of blood immediately evacuated by tube thoracostomy, bleeding at a rate of 150 mL/h to 200 mL/h for 2 to 4 hours, or persistent requirement for blood transfusion to maintain hemodynamic stability. The Eastern Association for the Surgery of Trauma recommendations state that patient physiology or chest tube output of 1500 mL in any 24-hour period should prompt operative management.[17] Incomplete drainage or retained hemothorax may lead to empyema and likely benefits from video-assisted thoracoscopy.

PNEUMOMEDIASTINUM
Background

Pneumomedisatinum (PM) is defined by the presence of air in the mediastinal space and may be spontaneous or traumatic. Spontaneous PM is characterized by a small air leak across a transalveolar pressure gradient. A transient increase in airway pressure causes alveolar rupture without pleural injury, and air dissects along the bronchovascular bundle into the mediastinum. This can occur from coughing or Valsalva maneuvers, in association with asthma or inhalational drug abuse, or without any identifiable cause at all.[31] In sports, spontaneous PM has been described in scuba diving,[32,33] weightlifting,[34] running,[35] and other athletic endeavors. It is generally self-limited, follows a benign course, and resolves quickly and uneventfully.[36] PM has also been reported as a result of trauma in collision sports, such as football[37] and ice hockey.[3,38] Heightened concern exists about traumatic PM because it suggests possible injury to the tracheobronchial tree or aeordigestive tract.[31] Olson,[38] however, proposed that PM in collision sports is related more closely to the spontaneous form than to PM in major trauma. It is reasonable to believe that a Valsalva-type force occurs during collision and produces alveolar rupture instead of tracheobronchial injury. He examined all cases of PM in the medical literature associated with collision sports from 1970 to 2010. The absence of complications in these cases lends truth to his assertion and has implications for management of PM in sports.

Diagnosis and Management

Chest pain, dyspnea, and neck pain are the most common symptoms of pneumomediastinum. Chest pain may radiate to the back or neck and worsen with inspiration or swallowing. Dysphonia, dysphagia, cough, and fever have also been reported.[31,38] Subcutaneous emphysema, usually in the neck or supraclavicular region, is frequently described because air can track from the mediastinum into the cervical fascial planes. Auscultatory findings include the Hamman crunch, in which crackles or a crunching sound is heard with each heartbeat. PM is diagnosed on a chest radiograph by air streaks in the superior mediastinum, prominence of the left cardiac silhouette, or subcutaneous emphysema in the neck.[31] Careful inspection for a continuous diaphragm sign, in which the diaphragm appears continuous across the entire thorax due to the presence of air, may also be a clue to PM (**Fig. 3**).

The greatest concern in the evaluation of anyone presenting with traumatic PM is for tracheobronchial or aerodigestive tract injury.[31] These injuries are rare but potentially fatal. Although 65% of blunt aerodigestive injuries present with PM and have 19% mortality, they occur in less than 0.1% of patients with blunt trauma. Additionally, almost 80% of patients with tracheobronchial injury die before reaching the hospital.[39] Boerhaave syndrome, or esophageal perforation, should be considered in any patient with PM after vomiting. It may present in similar fashion to spontaneous PM but progresses over several hours into a life-threatening condition, including shock. CT scan is recommended if esophageal perforation is suspected, because it may show characteristic findings of esophageal wall edema and thickening or esophageal fluid distention with adjacent air bubbles.[40] Water-soluble or barium contrast esophagram offers

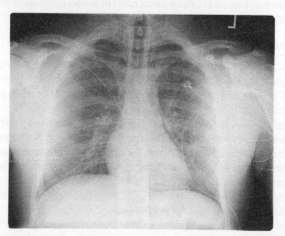

Fig. 3. Chest radiograph demonstrating the continuous diaphragm sign related to pneumomediastinum. Notice the continuity of the diaphragm across the entire thorax. (*Courtesy of* Robert Tubbs, MD, Providence, RI.)

confirmation when extravasation of contrast is present. CT is further useful in identification of occult PM and characterization of associated traumatic injuries, such as occult pneumothorax. Occult PM visualized on CT occurs in 6% of blunt chest trauma patients and is not associated with injury to the aeordigestive tract or increased mortality.[39]

Symptoms of PM should resolve within a few days, and radiographic resolution occurs between a few hours and 1 and 2 weeks.[31,38,39] Due to the benign course of spontaneous PM, a brief period of observation in the emergency department is usually all that is necessary to ensure stability. This observation period should be sufficient to distinguish clinically insignificant injury from more severe conditions that can lead to rapid deterioration, such as esophageal perforation.

Return to Play

As with the other conditions discussed in this article, there are no evidence-based guidelines to direct return-to-play decisions after pneumomediastinum. Return to activity is generally allowed once an athlete is asymptomatic and radiographic resolution has been documented. Cases in the literature support return to full participation between 1 and 4 weeks.[37,38] Olson[38] comments that PM in collision sports is a variant of spontaneous PM and return to sports can likely occur in 2 weeks or less. Other injuries, such as concomitant pneumothorax, may delay the return to sports. Recommendations regarding air travel are similar to those of pneumothorax.[24] Air travel is presumed safe at 2 to 3 weeks, with the understanding that radiographic resolution of PM has occurred.

PULMONARY CONTUSION
Background

Pulmonary contusion is the most common complication of blunt chest injury,[41] typically resulting from high-energy trauma, such as motor vehicle crashes and falls. It is characterized by parenchymal hemorrhage, interstitial edema, and alveolar collapse, all potentially leading to compromised respiratory function.[42] It is rarely reported in association with sports participation, but a few case reports in football players exist in the literature.[43,44] One case of pulmonary contusion in a diver has also been reported as a result of impacting the water awkwardly.[45]

Diagnosis and Management

Clinical and radiographic manifestations of pulmonary contusion may present immediately or in a delayed fashion. Typical findings include dyspnea and hypoxemia; tachypnea, hemoptysis, chest pain, and wheezing may also occur.[43] Auscultation of the lungs might reveal crackles or diminished breath sounds. Common to all cases of thoracic trauma, conventional CXR is the initial imaging study of choice. The size of the contusion, however, is often underestimated on the initial CXR and findings may be absent altogether in 10% to 36% of cases.[41,46–48] Focal or diffuse opacification extending beyond lung segments or lobes is diagnostic in the appropriate clinical setting, and these findings may develop up to 48 hours after injury.[49]

CT has improved sensitivity over CXR for detection of pulmonary contusion.[50] Because it has added value in quantifying the injury, CT is often cited as the preferred imaging modality.[41] The clinical significance of contusions identified by CT has been questioned, however, and may not alter management. Deunk and colleagues[50] studied the implications and outcomes of occult pulmonary contusion. They reported on 98 patients with pulmonary contusion identified by both CXR and CT compared with

157 patients demonstrating occult pulmonary contusion visualized on CT only. They concluded that outcomes in patients with occult pulmonary contusion are similar to those without lung injury and better than those with findings on CXR and CT.

Management of pulmonary contusion depends on the extent of injury. Care of minor injuries, such as those associated with sports, is supportive and includes supplemental oxygen, pain management, pulmonary toilet, hemodynamic monitoring, and judicious administration of intravenous fluids.[42,49] The administration of crystalloid has been thought to worsen hypoxia in pulmonary contusion, but this has not been supported in the literature.[49] Mechanical ventilation may be necessary in cases of severe hypoxemia. There is no role for empiric antibiotics in pulmonary contusion.

Complications of pulmonary contusion range from pneumonia to acute respiratory distress syndrome and are associated with more severe injury and greater than 20% contusion. Mortality approaches 25% in those that develop acute respiratory distress syndrome.[41] Other clinical variables predisposing to poor outcome are pulmonary contusion on admission CXR, 3 or more rib fractures, chest insertion and drainage, and hypoxia (Pao_2/Fio_2 <250) on admission. Injuries reported in athletes are minor by comparison, and isolated pulmonary contusion in young, healthy individuals is not associated with mortality.[48]

Return to Play

There are no specific data to guide return to play for athletes after pulmonary contusion. Each of the cases reported in football players involved occult, mildly symptomatic contusions identified by CT.[43,44] All athletes returned to exercise within 2 to 3 days and were cleared for full participation 1 week after injury without recurrence of symptoms or adverse outcome. This is consistent with the general understanding that uncomplicated pulmonary contusions resolve within approximately 7 days.[42] Two players returned to football with a flack jacket for added protection, although there is no evidence to support this practice. Although chest wall pain may persist for several weeks, persistent respiratory symptoms should preclude a return to activity.

SUMMARY

Pulmonary injury from blunt thoracic trauma is uncommon during athletic participation. Experience with traumatic pneumothorax, hemothorax, and pulmonary contusion is derived primarily from the trauma literature and represents injury severity and mechanisms that may be substantially different from those found in sports. Pneumomediastinum in collision sports, however, seems closely related to the spontaneous entity. Although general principles for management of each of these conditions are well understood, return-to-play guidelines are based largely on opinion, case reports, and common sense. More experience with these injuries may help to better define recommendations for specific management strategies in athletes and return to competition.

REFERENCES

1. Stahel PF, Smith WR, Moore EE. Current trends in resuscitation strategy for the multiply injured patient. Injury 2009;40(Suppl 4):S27–35.
2. Sharma A, Jindal P. Principles of diagnosis and management of traumatic pneumothorax. J Emerg Trauma Shock 2008;1(1):34–41.
3. Partridge RA, Coley A, Bowie R, et al. Sports-related pneumothorax. Ann Emerg Med 1997;30:539–41.
4. Levy AS, Bassett F, Lintner S, et al. Pulmonary barotraumas: diagnosis in American football players. Three cases in three years. Am J Sports Med 1996;24:227–9.

5. Soundappan SV, Holland AJ, Browne G. Sports-related pneumothorax in children. Pediatr Emerg Care 2005;21(4):259–60.
6. Sadat-Ali M, Al-Arfaj AL, Mohanna M. Pneumothorax due to soccer injury [letter]. Br J Sports Med 1986;20:91.
7. Salahuddin M, James LA, Bass ES. SCUBA medicine: a first-responder's guide to diving injuries. Curr Sports Med Rep 2011;10(3):134–9.
8. Marnejon T, Sarac S, Cropp AJ. Spontaneous pneumothorax in weightlifters. J Sports Med Phys Fitness 1995;35(2):124–6.
9. Kizer KW, MacQuarrie MB. Pulmonary air leaks resulting from outdoor sports: a clinical series and literature review. Am J Sports Med 1999;27(4):517–20.
10. Milne LW. Thoracic trauma in polo: two cases and a review of the literature. J Emerg Med 2011;40(4):410–4.
11. Putukian M. Pneumothorax and pneumomediastinum. Clin Sports Med 2004;23: 443–54.
12. Wilkerson RG, Stone MB. Sensitivity of bedside ultrasound and supine anteroposterior chest radiographs for the identification of pneumothorax after blunt trauma. Acad Emerg Med 2010;17(1):11–7.
13. Sangster GP, Gonzalez-Beicos A, Carbo AI. Blunt traumatic injuries of the lung parenchyma, pleura, thoracic wall, and intrathoracic airways: multidetector computed tomography imaging findings. Emerg Radiol 2007;14:297–310.
14. Ball CG, Kirkpatrick AW, Laupland KB, et al. Incidence, risk factors, and outcomes for occult pneumothoraces in victims of major trauma. J Trauma 2005;59:917–25.
15. Gordon R. The deep sulcus sign. Radiology 1980;136(1):25–7.
16. Yadav K, Jalili M, Zehtabchi S. Management of traumatic occult pneumothorax. Resuscitation 2010;81:1063–8.
17. Mowery NT, Gunter OL, Collier BR, et al. Practice management guidelines for management of hemothorax and occult pneumothorax. J Trauma 2011;70(2): 510–8.
18. Baumann MH, Strange C, Heffner JE, et al. Management of spontaneous pneumothorax: an American College of Chest Physicians Delphi consensus statement. Chest 2001;119:590–602.
19. Symington L, McGugan E. Towards evidence based emergency medicine: best BETs from the Manchester Royal Infirmary. Is a chest drain necessary in stable patients with traumatic pneumothorax? Emerg Med J 2008;25(7):439–40.
20. Obeid FN, Shapiro MJ, Richardson HH, et al. Catheter aspiration for simple pneumothorax (CASP) in the outpatient management of simple traumatic pneumothorax. J Trauma 1985;25(9):882–6.
21. Vallee P, Sullivan M, Richardson H, et al. Sequential treatment of a simple pneumothorax. Ann Emerg Med 1988;17(9):936–42.
22. Chan SS. The role of simple aspiration in the management of primary spontaneous pneumothorax. J Emerg Med 2008;34(2):131–8.
23. Amaral JF. Thoracoabdominal injuries in the athlete. Clin Sports Med 1997;16(4): 739–53.
24. Aerospace Medical Association Medical Guidelines Task Force. Medical guidelines for airline travel, 2nd ed. Aviat Space Environ Med 2003;74(Suppl 5):A1–19.
25. Cheatham ML, Safcsak K. Air travel following traumatic pneumothorax: when is it safe? Am Surg 1999;65(12):1160–4.
26. Watanabe M, Igarashi N, Naruke M, et al. Traumatic pulmonary pseudocyst with hemopneumothorax in a football player. Clin J Sport Med 2005;15:41–3.
27. Schneider V, Bratzke H. Traumatic rupture of the aorta after a jump from the 3-meter-board. Z Rechtsmed 1979;83(2):169–77 [in German].

28. Shimizu K, Ogura H, Nakagawa Y, et al. Lethal aortic arch injury caused by a rugby tackle: a case report. Am J Sports Med 2008;36(8):1611–4.
29. Buchman TG, Hall BL, Bowling WM, et al. Thoracic trauma. In: Tintinalli JE, Kelen GD, Stapczynski JS, editors. Emergency medicine: a comprehensive study guide. New York: McGraw-Hill; 2004. p. 1595–613.
30. Bilello JF, Davis JW, Lemaster DM. Occult traumatic hemothorax: where can sleeping dogs lie? Am J Surg 2005;190:841–4.
31. Takada K, Matsumoto S, Hiramatsu T, et al. Spontaneous pneumomediastinum: an algorithm for diagnosis and management. Ther Adv Respir Dis 2009;3:301–7.
32. Cheung HY, Law S, Wong KH, et al. Spontaneous pneumomediastinum in a scuba diver. Hong Kong Med J 2006;12(2):152–3.
33. Kosaka T, Haraguchi M, Tsuneoka N, et al. Spontaneous pneumomediastinumn as a result of SCUBA diving. Eur J Emerg Med 2007;14(2):118–9.
34. Asplund CA, Howard TM, O'Connor FG. Spontaneous pneumomediastinum in a weightlifter. Curr Sports Med Rep 2003;2(2):63–4.
35. Townes DA. Spontaneous pneumomediastinum in a marathon runner. Br J Sports Med 2006;40(10):878–9.
36. Mihos P, Potaris K, Gakidis I, et al. Sports-related spontaneous pneumomediastinum. Ann Thorac Surg 2004;78:983–6.
37. Dyste KH, Newkirk KM. Pneumomediastinum in a high school football player: a case report. J Athl Train 1998;33(4):362–4.
38. Olson RP. Return to collision sport after pneumomediastinum. Curr Sports Med Rep 2012;11(2):58–63.
39. Rezende-Neto JB, Hoffmann J, Al Mahroos M, et al. Occult pneumomediastinum in blunt chest trauma: clinical significance. Injury 2010;41:40–3.
40. de Lutio di Castelguidone E, Merola S, Pinto A. Esophageal injuries: spectrum of multidetector row CT findings. Eur J Radiol 2006;59(3):344–8.
41. Miller PR, Croce MA, Bee TK, et al. ARDS after pulmonary contusion: accurate measurement of contusion volume identifies high-risk patients. J Trauma 2001; 51(2):223–30.
42. Cohn SM. Pulmonary contusion: review of the clinical entity. J Trauma 1997;42: 973–9.
43. Lively MW, Stone D. Pulmonary contusion in football players. Clin J Sport Med 2006;16:177–8.
44. Meese MA, Sebastianelli WJ. Pumonary contusion secondary to blunt trauma in a collegiate football player. Clin J Sport Med 1997;7:309–10.
45. Lively MW. Pulmonary contusion in a collegiate diver: a case report. J Med Case Rep 2011;10(5):362.
46. Tyburski JG, Collinge JD, Wilson RF, et al. Pulmonary contusion: quantifying the lesions on chest x-ray films and the factors affecting prognosis. J Trauma 1999;46(5):833–8.
47. Schild HH, Strunk H, Weber W, et al. Pulmonary contusion. CT vs. plain radiograms. J Comput Assist Tomogr 1989;13(3):417.
48. Hoff SJ, Shotts SD, Eddy VA, et al. Outcome of isolated pulmonary contusion in blunt trauma patients. Am Surg 1994;60(2):138–42.
49. Wanek S, Mayberry JC. Blunt thoracic trauma: flail chest, pulmonary contusion, and blast injury. Crit Care Clin 2004;20:71–81.
50. Deunk J, Poels TC, Brink M, et al. The clinical outcome of occult pulmonary contusion on multidetector-row computed tomography in blunt trauma patients. J Trauma 2010;68:387–94.

Blunt Cardiac Contusions

Melissa Mascaro, MD[a],*, Thomas H. Trojian, MD[b]

KEYWORDS

- Cardiac injury • Blunt cardiac trauma • Commotio cordis • Sudden collapse
- Chest wall protectors

KEY POINTS

- Nonpenetrating cardiac injury can include hemothorax, pneumothorax, pulmonary contusion, and rib or sternal fractures.
- Spectrum of injury varies from contused myocardium to cardiac rupture.
- It becomes worrisome if chest is struck at a vulnerable point in the cardiac cycle just before the peak of the T wave.
- Watch for brief periods of consciousness followed by sudden collapse and ventricular fibrillation.
- Prevention theories include softer balls used in sports, such as baseball, and chest wall protectors in contact sports that cover the left chest wall and precordium.
- Return-to-play guidelines are most often left to a clinician's best judgment.

INTRODUCTION

The term, *blunt cardiac contusion* (BCC), formerly known as myocardial contusion, has acquired its name from its description as a nonpenetrating cardiac injury. The spectrum of injury varies from contused myocardium, showing muscle necrosis, edema, and hemorrhagic infiltrate, to cardiac rupture.

Physicians are concerned about the spectrum of outcomes, which vary from asymptomatic changes on an ECG to cardiogenic shock and sudden death. With no standard diagnostic criteria, the true incidence remains unclear. There is no current gold standard in diagnosis; however, all patients who have a clinical history and an altered cardiac function must be considered as patients with BCC. Unlike adults, children with blunt cardiac injuries (BCIs) have few presenting signs and symptoms. Children are believed more susceptible because of the elasticity and compressibility of their chest walls.[1] Monitoring is crucial because problems often evolve over time.

Funding Sources: The author has nothing to disclose.
Conflict of Interest: Nil.
[a] Department of Sports Medicine, St Francis Hospital, University of Connecticut, 99 Woodland Street, Hartford, CT 06105, USA; [b] Director of Injury Prevention and Sports Outreach, Team, Physician University of Connecticut
* Corresponding author.
E-mail address: Mmascaro@stfranciscare.org

One of the more common cardiac contusion fears in the sports world is the development of commotio cordis. It was first distinguished from bruising of the heart, or contusio cordis, in 1763. Commotio cordis is differentiated from cardiac contusion (contusio cordis), a situation in which blunt chest trauma causes structural cardiac damage, such as that observed in motor vehicular accidents.[2] First described in 1857, the term, *commotio cordis*, translates as *disturbance of the heart* and refers to cardiac concussion in the absence of injury.[1]

BCI is typically found in patients who are struck in the pericardium at a vulnerable point in the cardiac cycle just before the peak of the T wave. The impact usually results in ventricular fibrillation; however, there are several other rhythms that have been found to occur as a result of BCI, including ventricular tachycardia, bradyarrythmias, idioventricular arrythmias, complete heart block, and asystole.[1] There is usually no underlying cardiac disease found in these patients. This is common in sports that have projectile objects that can hit the chest, such as baseball, lacrosse, ice hockey, shadow boxing, and martial arts.

Estimates of the impact velocity of baseballs causing commotio cordis range from 20 to 50 miles per hour.[3] There has been some evidence that softer objects can help prevent this type of injury and further research should be done to evaluate.[4]

ANATOMY/PATHOPHYSIOLOGY

The right ventricle is the most common site of BCC, most likely secondary to the anterior location of the right atrium and ventricle within the mediastinum. There has been concurrent injury to more than 1 chamber in more than 50% of BCC patients.[5] Additional chest injuries that can occur with myocardial contusion include hemothorax, pneumothorax, pulmonary contusion, and rib or sternal fractures. Physicians should remember to evaluate for these types of injuries when presented with patients who have a history consistent with BCC.

MECHANISM OF INJURY

BCC arises from a variety of mechanisms, including

1. Direct precordial impact
2. Crush injury resulting from compression between the sternum and spine
3. Deceleration or torsion causing a tear in the heart at a point of fixation

PATIENT PRESENTATION

When viewing from the sideline, physicians must have a focused eye to know which player to watch when there is more than one player on the field. Remember that a player who is hit in the chest by either a ball or a person is at highest risk. This is true even if the blow is innocent in appearance. Brief periods of consciousness are followed by sudden collapse and ventricular fibrillation. When covering a sporting event that has a projectile object, it is crucial to prepare for worst-case scenarios that cause life-threatening injuries. If a blunt chest injury is witnessed and a player has a brief period of consciousness followed by sudden collapse, one attempt at defibrillation should be followed by immediate cardiopulmonary resuscitation.[6]

Patients who are hit in the chest but do not collapse often present with chest pain or discomfort. Pain may or may not be anginal in nature. There may be associated dyspnea, flail chest, ecchymosis, and sternal fractures seen on clinical examination. In blunt thoracic trauma, cardiac arrythmias, a new murmur, heart failure, or hypotension can signal cardiac injury.[7] It is also important to note any medications a patient may be taking, which may mask tachycardia.

MANAGEMENT

After a history of BCI, all patients should undergo a physical examination with emphasis on vital signs, head and neck, lungs, and heart once patients are stabilized. Caution should be taken if jugular venous distention, hypotension, tenderness of the chest, ecchymosis, distant heart sounds, or murmurs are found.[8] Rapid deterioration can occur.

All patients suspected of having a BCC should begin by having a 12-lead ECG obtained; however this is not pathognomic. In adults, nonspecific ECG changes are common and a thorough clinical history should be used. Most changes on ECG are noted within 24 hours after suspected injury.[5] In children, sinus tachycardia, ST-T wave abnormalities, low-voltage QRS abnormalities, heart block, premature ventricular contractions, junctional rhythms, and ventricular tachycardia may be found.[4]

The next step in evaluating BCIs is a chest radiograph. This helps in diagnosing rib fractures, pneumothorax, and widening of the mediastinum. All patients should be observed in a unit that is capable of handling hemodynamically unstable patients in the event that hypotension develops or there is evidence of cardiac dysfunction.

A focused abdominal sonogram for trauma scan may be performed if a patient presents to an emergency department. This may help in determining if pericardial fluid exists and a cardiac tampanode is developing.

Cardiac enzymes, such as creatine kinase and creatine kinase–MB, were used initially to evaluate for BCCs but, with little specificity, they were abandoned. Instead, cardiac troponin I (cTnI) has been used to screen for BCCs. The specificity of both cTnI and cardiac troponin T (cTnT) for BCCs is greater than that for creatine kinase and creatine kinase–MB, because neither cTnI nor cTnT is released with skeletal muscle injury.

The value of cTnI increases when combined with admission ECG findings, as reported by Schultz and colleagues.[5] In this study, the sensitivity of abnormal ECG findings with serial normal cTnI increases. A diagnosis of BCC should be supported by elevated serum cTnI and cTnT as well as additional clinical data.

Newer studies continue to find improvements in troponin testing characteristics. A normal troponin I at 4 to 6 hours after trauma could rule out BCI in a hemodynamically healthy patient. There are other studies that reveal a normal troponin I has a negative predictive value of 93% to 94% for BCI patients. By using a combination of a normal ECG with a normal troponin I, the negative predictive value can be increased to 100%.[9]

Echocardiography is a useful tool to assess cardiac function and diagnosis of noncardiac injuries, such as pericardial effusion or myocardial rupture, but it has little use as a screening tool.[5]

Other cardiac imaging tests, such as radionucleotide angiography, technetium Tc 99 m scintigraphy, single-photon emission CT scans, and thallium Tl 201 scintigraphy, may be used to evaluate for further damage caused by blunt cardiac trauma; however, there has been no evidence for any of these modalities used as diagnostic tools.[5]

If a complete work-up is obtained, patients not at risk could potentially be discharged from the hospital with appropriate follow-up (**Fig. 1**).

RETURN-TO-PLAY GUIDELINES

There are currently no standard return-to-play guidelines for BCI. This should be a source for further research; however, physicians should use good judgment and consider athletes' mental and physical readiness to return to play.

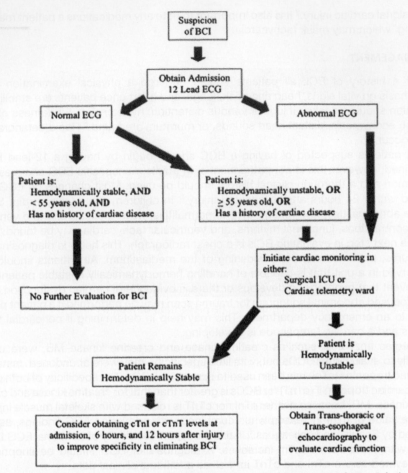

Fig. 1. Algorithm for the evaluation of patients suspected of having BCI. (*From* Schultz JM, Trunkey DD. Blunt cardiac injury. Crit Care Clin 2004;20(1):57–70; with permission.)

Only a few studies have evaluated the long-term effects of BCI. Stuartis and colleagues[7] evaluated 44 patients who had sustained a traumatic myocardial contusion. These patients were compared with a control cohort of patients matched for injury severity without cardiac injury. At follow-up, 13 patients with BCI were indistinguishable from a control group of 12 patients, according to the New York Heart Association classification. Left and right ventricular ejection fractions were similar at rest and under exercise conditions in these 2 groups of patients. The investigators concluded that traumatic BCI of the left or right ventricle usually resolves without significant functional sequelae within 1 year of injury.

SUMMARY

The absence of a clear definition and accepted gold standard for testing makes the diagnosis of cardiac contusion difficult. Nonpenetrating cardiac injuries, known as blunt cardiac trauma, vary in severity from contused myocardium, showing muscle necrosis, edema, and hemorrhagic infiltrate, to cardiac rupture. In those sports in which there is no solid, hard ball, impacts with elbows, fists, and helmets are also a cause of concern. Commotio cordis is reported in activities of daily living in which impact to the chest wall occurs with fists or other hard compact objects. Physicians covering sporting events should be aware that blunt trauma injuries to the chest can lead to death if not treated promptly.

Prevention theories include using softer balls in sports, such as baseball, and chest wall protectors in contact sports that cover the left chest wall and precordium.

Future directions for improving the diagnosis and management of blunt thoracic trauma involve diagnostic testing, endovascular techniques, and patient selection. The implementation of prompt cardiopulmonary resuscitation and prehospital automatic external defibrillator use has been shown to increase survival rates.[10] The survival rate is approximately 15% to begin with and, with every minute defibrillation is delayed, survival declines 7% to 10%.[6] Return-to-play guidelines are most often left to a clinician's best judgment because there is a lack of data in the community.

REFERENCES

1. Marshall DT, Gilbert JD, Byard RW. The spectrum of findings in cases of sudden death due to blunt cardiac trauma—'commotio cordis'. Am J Forensic Med Pathol 2008;29(1):1–4.
2. Link MS. Commotio cordis: ventricular fibrillation triggered by chest impact-induced abnormalities in repolarization. Circ Arrhythm Electrophysiol 2012;5(2):425–32.
3. Link MS, Maron BJ, Wang PJ, et al. Reduced risk of sudden death from chest wall blows (commotio cordis) with safety baseballs. Pediatrics 2002;109(5):873–7.
4. Gunjan K. Management of pediatric cardiac trauma in the ED. Clinical Pediatric Emergency Medicine 2011;12(4):323–31.
5. Schultz JM, Trunkey DD. Blunt cardiac injury. Crit Care Clin 2004;20(1):57–70.
6. Salib EA, Cyran SE, Cilley RE, et al. Efficacy of bystander cardiopulmonary resuscitation and out-of-hospital automated external defibrillation as life-saving therapy in commotio cordis. J Pediatr 2005;147(6):863–6.
7. Stuartis M, McCallum D, Sutherland G, et al. Lack of significant long-term sequelae following traumatic myocardial contusion. Arch Intern Med 1986;146(9):1765–9.
8. Elie MC. Blunt cardiac injury. Mt Sinai J Med 2006;73(2):542–52.
9. Collins JN, Cole FJ, Weireter LJ, et al. The usefulness of serum troponin levels in evaluating cardiac injury. Am Surg 2001;67(9):821–5 [discussion: 825–6].
10. Zangwill SD, Strasburger JF. Commotio cordis. Pediatr Clin North Am 2004;51(5):1347–54.

Closed Head Injury

Hamish A. Kerr, MD, MSc

KEYWORDS

- Concussion • Intracranial hemorrhage • Skull fracture • Facial fracture • Eye injuries
- Scalp laceration • Pinna hematoma

KEY POINTS

- At least 3% of sports-related injuries are to the head, making this a relatively common injury.
- Head injuries vary from the very minor laceration to the life-threatening intracranial hemorrhage.
- A high index of suspicion and conducting serial examination will often help differentiate the more serious head injured athlete.

The human head is designed to help one avoid trauma, with sensory input from the eyes and ears, and a position at the apex of the skeleton. Nonetheless, participation in the sporting arena can put the head at risk. Head injuries are often some of the most concerning events witnessed while covering contact/collision sports. There is a spectrum of severity, from relatively benign soft tissue superficial damage, to bleeding and tearing of the brain. This article will discuss closed head trauma and outline specific injuries to the face, brain, skull, and its surroundings.

EPIDEMIOLOGY OF CLOSED HEAD INJURY

It has been estimated that 3% of all sport-related injuries are to the head,[1] with an increasing percentage seen with age:

- 2.8% sports-related injuries in children younger than 10 years
- 3.7% of sports-related injuries in 10- to 14-year old children
- 4.2% of sports-related injuries in 15- to 19-year-olds

Head injuries are 1 of the top 4 body areas injured (ankle, knee, shoulder, head) in contact sports such as rugby.[2,3] In soccer, estimates suggest 4% to 22% of all injuries

Disclosures: None.
Conflict of Interest: None.
Primary Care Sports Medicine Fellowship, Division Internal Medicine/Pediatrics, Albany Medical College, 724 Watervliet-Shaker Road, Latham, NY 12110, USA
E-mail address: kerrh@mail.amc.edu

Clin Sports Med 32 (2013) 273–287
http://dx.doi.org/10.1016/j.csm.2012.12.008
0278-5919/13/$ – see front matter © 2013 Elsevier Inc. All rights reserved.

are to the head.[4,5] They are common in winter sports,[6] although the introduction of helmets for skiing and snowboarding has certainly diminished the risk of more severe head injury.[7] Other helmeted sports such as football, ice hockey and men's lacrosse still have a risk of functional brain injury despite the protective equipment.[8,9] Protective equipment is also recommended in projectile sports such as baseball and cricket for certain positions are at risk of being hit by the ball.[7] Baseball causes the most eye injuries in 5- to 15-year-old children in the United States, while in 25- to 65-year-olds, racquet sports cause the most eye injuries.[10–12] Prevention is possible with appropriate eyewear.[13]

Closed-head injuries vary in severity from minor scrapes, lacerations, and abrasions that are inherent to almost every game of rugby, to the most severe brain injuries including intracranial hemorrhage, which has a significant mortality rate.[14,15] Differentiating the minor from the most severe can be difficult, may not immediately be apparent to even the highly trained and experienced physician, and often requires longitudinal reassessment to identify the athlete who is deteriorating.

CLOSED-HEAD INJURY INITIAL EVALUATION

Fieldside evaluation of a witnessed closed-head injury begins with the assumption of cervical spine injury and possible spinal cord injury in any athlete knocked unconscious.[14,16–19] Airway, breathing, and circulation must be assessed before evaluation of head itself. If there is a dilated pupil, endotracheal intubation can be considered before transport on a spinal board.

Although some injuries such as a bleeding laceration may be obvious immediately, brain injury, and concussion in particular, may take careful examination to exclude. In the absence of a loss of consciousness, an athlete should be removed from the field of play and assessed on the sideline. Glasgow Coma Scale (GCS) and Maddocks questions can help assess consciousness and orientation and are included in the Sports Concussion Assessment Tool Version 2 (SCAT II) that was developed for this purpose.[20–23] Deterioration in scoring on serial SCAT II assessment, scoring greater than13 on the GCS, or any focal neurologic finding should prompt urgent transport to a trauma center.[14,24]

Management of specific injuries identified on secondary survey is discussed in the following sections.

SOFT TISSUE TRAUMA: SCALP AND FACIAL LACERATIONS

Lacerations should be irrigated with sterile saline and explored for foreign bodies or underlying damage. Pressure should be applied to control bleeding. Sutures are required to close the wound. Tetanus prophylaxis is advised. Simple lacerations less than 4 cm that are not at points of high skin tension are recommended to be closed by a tissue adhesive, such as Dermabond (Ethicon, Inc. Menlo Park, CA),[25] which showed superior cosmetic outcome without increased complications in a randomized trial versus sutures.

Deep absorbable sutures are necessary if there is separation of deep tissue. With lacerations over an area of dynamic muscle contraction (eg, forehead, perioral, or over the mandible), initial subcutaneous sutures can decrease wound tension.[25,26] An invisible soft tissue surface or scalp laceration can be closed with 5-0 sutures,[27] while facial lacerations should be closed with 7-0 monofilament nylon sutures. Lacerations involving the lacrimal apparatus, parotid gland, facial nerve (facial droop or asymmetry), or anatomic borders should be referred, as should those across structural or functional borders such as vermilion border of lip, eyelid, nasal alar rims, or helical rims of ear, which require great precision in the repair to prevent poor cosmetic results.

SOFT TISSUE TRAUMA: FACIAL SKIN ABRASION

Abrasions should be cleaned with antimicrobial soap and water, then irrigated with sterile saline. Topical anesthetic is appropriate before cleaning larger abrasions. All debris should be removed from the abrasion, or tattooing will occur. Tetanus prophylaxis is again necessary.

SOFT TISSUE TRAUMA: PINNA HEMATOMA

Trauma to the pinna is relatively common in collision sports where participants do not wear helmets. Rugby is perhaps the best example; pinna hematomas are the rugby team physician's bread and butter. Hematomas are best drained in the days after the injury,; then silicone mold material should be placed in the same area to prevent reaccumulation.[28–30] Rugby players can help prevent pinna hematomas by taping their ears or by wearing a scrum cap.[31]

FACIAL TRAUMA: EYE INJURY

Evaluation of a possible eye injury (not always possible fieldside) should include[32]

- Assessment of visual acuity (eg, handheld eye chart)
- Gross external examination (inspection and palpation of globes, swelling, orbital rim step-off)
- Fundoscopy
- Optic nerve function
- Pupils (size, reactivity, perception of brightness)
- Visual fields and external ocular muscle function
- Intraocular pressure[33]

EYE INJURY: VISION-THREATENING INJURIES

Injuries to the globe, retrobulbar hemorrhage, traumatic optic neuropathy, and eyelid laceration can all result in loss of vision if not identified and managed appropriately.[34] A relative afferent papillary defect (RAPD) is a sensitive indicator of visual impairment suggesting asymmetrical damage to retina, optic nerve, chiasm, or optic tract.

Globe Rupture

Globe rupture is differentiated into open, with a full-thickness tear through cornea, and sclera and closed, without a full-thickness tear. Globe rupture is a common cause of blindness after trauma; it requires a high index of suspicion, as it is not always obvious.[35] Signs of globe rupture include decreased visual acuity, a severe subconjunctival hemorrhage involving all quadrants of the conjunctiva, and limited external ocular muscle movement. In addition, globe collapse may be seen manifested by low intraocular pressure (IOP), extruded eye contents, and a hyphema if open. In this circumstance, applied pressure can cause further expulsion of globe if there is an open rupture, and this should be avoided at all cost. A shield should be taped over the eye and the patient transported to a facility where surgery can be accomplished within 24 hours.

Retrobulbar Hemorrhage

This condition is a compartment syndrome of the eye, with irreversible damage occurring after 60 minutes of ischemia.[36] Hemorrhage and edema in the orbit lead to an increase in IOP, compression of the blood supply, and ischemia of optic nerve and retina. Signs of retrobulbar hemorrhage include proptosis, loss of vision, pain, and an absent RAPD or dilated pupil. The condition requires relief of the pressure with a lateral canthotomy and inferior cantholysis, then ultimately surgical decompression.

Traumatic Optic Neuropathy

Force transmitted to the optic canal, thus injuring the optic nerve, can result in loss of vision. It is perhaps best avoided with appropriate eyewear rather than being amenable to acute management.

Eyelid Laceration

Eyelid laceration may be a sign of a more serious ocular injury. An assessment for a penetrating globe injury or foreign body should be conducted. If the eyelid cannot close, the cornea dries, so even small eyelid lacerations can threaten vision loss. Medial lacerations can damage the lacrimal system, and upper eyelid laceration can damage the levator palpebrae, resulting in ptosis.[27] Eyelid lacerations should be treated with generous antibiotic ointment application, covering with a wet gauze, and then surgical repair.

FACIAL TRAUMA: DENTAL INJURIES

An avulsed tooth should be replaced in its socket whenever possible, and the athlete instructed to bite down on some gauze to keep it in place. If replacement is not possible, the tooth should be placed in Hank's solution to preserve it.[37–40] The tooth should be handled only by the crown and gently washed if not clean. Reimplantation within 30 minutes results in a 90% success rate, saving the tooth, so an immediate dental referral is essential. A delay greater than 2 hours decreases the success rate to only a 5% chance.[41] Mouth guards are a key prevention strategy for dental injuries.[42]

FACIAL TRAUMA: FACIAL FRACTURE

Facial fractures account for 4% to 18% of all sports injuries, and sports are responsible for 6% to 33% of all facial bone fractures.[43–45] Midface and mandibular fractures may threaten the airway or can cause a lot of bleeding. Orbital or zygomatic fractures can threaten vision.

Facial Fracture: Orbital Blowout Fracture

Orbital blowout fractures generally result from blunt trauma to eye, and then collapse of the inferior or medial orbital wall. The collapse may entrap the medial and lateral rectus muscles, thus reducing external ocular muscle movement on examination. Orbital blowout fractures are more common than globe rupture, as the collapse of the inferior orbital wall helps decrease the amount of pressure absorbed by the globe.[46] Physical examination often reveals diplopia, enopthalmos, and infraorbital hypoesthesia secondary to damage to the infraorbital nerve.[47,48] Computed tomography (CT) scan imaging can exclude strangulation of the extraocular muscle, which can otherwise cause necrosis if not identified.

Superior orbital fissure syndrome occurs when there is compression of cranial nerves 3 or 4 as they pass through the superior orbital fissure. Typically, the increased IOP will limit external ocular muscle movement and cause paresthesiae of the forehead and brow. This syndrome needs emergency surgery (**Fig. 1**).[49]

Facial Fracture: Zygomatic Fractures

Zygomatic anatomy includes the cheekbone, orbit, and orbital rim. The zygomatic bone acts as an attachment for the masseter muscle and the outer facial frame. Zygomatic fracture therefore affects vision, jaw function, and the width of the face. Mechanism of injury is usually blunt trauma, presenting with flattening of the cheekbone. There may also be subconjunctival hemorrhage, periorbital ecchymosis, a palpable step-off in the upper outer or inferior orbital rim, emphysema, trismus, malposition of the globe, and diplopia. Fracture management should include operative fixation within 2 weeks[50,51] for displaced or comminuted fractures (**Fig. 2**).

Facial Fracture: Maxillary Fracture

Maxillary fractures were originally described by Le Fort in 1901 and are classified by the most superior level of the fracture site.[52] Maxillary fractures are usually very high-impact injuries. Le Fort II and Le Fort III are more severe and can cause airway compromise and require admission.[53] Reducing the fracture can help control bleeding and alleviate airway compromise (**Fig. 3**).

Facial Fracture: Nasal Fractures

The nose is the most commonly fractured bone in face (**Fig. 4**).[54]

Clinical presentation of nasal fracture frequently includes epistaxis from the capillary plexus in the anteroinferior septum. Initial management is to apply pressure, then consider nasal packing, and perhaps a nasal decongestant spray.[55] It is important

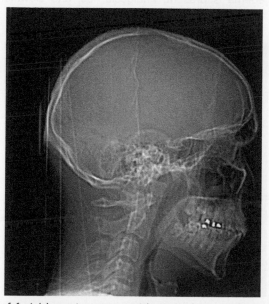

Fig. 1. Illustration of facial bones' anatomy with sagittal X-ray of a collegiate basketball player who sustained a contusion injury to his cheekbone. (*Courtesy of* Greg Dashnaw, Head Athletic Trainer, Siena College, Loudonville, NY.)

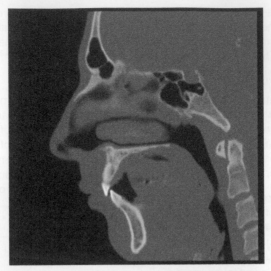

Fig. 2. Sagittal CT scan of face of basketball player with facial injury.

to identify previous surgery or deformity when making a decision regarding repair. After repair, the nose will return to a previously deformed shape if there was a previous untreated injury.[54] Examination of a nasal injury should include inspection of the septum for hematoma formation and drainage if present. Repeat examinations may be necessary to exclude a recurrence.

Performance of closed reduction should be conducted in the first few hours after a nasal fracture. After closed reduction 14% to 50% of patients still require rhinoplasty.[56] If facial edema is present, analgesia, ice, and elevation are warranted. Specialist referral is suggested within 5 to 7 days.[54]

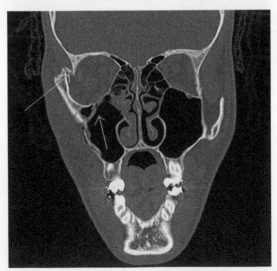

Fig. 3. Le Fort I fracture of the maxilla after patient struck by a baseball (right lateral orbital wall fracture, zygoma and right maxillary sinus fractures). (*Courtesy of* Lippincott Williams & Wilkins.)

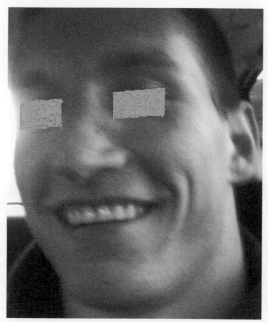

Fig. 4. International rugby player with a nasal fracture after sustaining an injury during a tackle.

Facial Fracture: Mandibular Fractures

A mandibular fracture is identified clinically by local swelling, malocclusion of the jaw, numbness in the lower lip, and intraoral lacerations. Malocclusion is best assessed by biting a tongue blade. Mandibular fractures are more often than not multiple; thus excluding a contralateral fracture is warranted. Frequency varies by location (condyle 30%, ramus 3%, angle 25%, body 25%, mental 15%). Tooth avulsion or intraoral bleeding can cause airway compromise, as can posterior displacement of the tongue with a bilateral mandible fracture of the body or angle.[57,58] CT scan imaging or Panorex imaging is preferred and referral to an oral maxillofacial surgeon for operative fixation (**Fig. 5**).

Roccia and colleagues[59] recommend a stepwise return to play after a facial fracture as follows

- No activity days 1 to 20
- Light aerobic days 21 to 30
- Noncontact days 31 to 40
- Afterday 41, full contact and game

Progress should occur if asymptomatic. In combat sports, return should not occur before 3 months. There are no evidence-based facemask guidelines for accomplishing an earlier return to play.

SKULL FRACTURE

Skull fractures are often associated with an underlying brain injury resulting clinically in a focal neurologic deficit or seizure.[14,60] Clinical assessment should also include inspection of the nares and external auditory meatus for clear fluid that could be

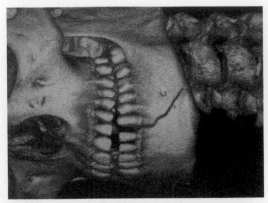

Fig. 5. International rugby player with mandibular fracture sustained during a tournament.

cerebrospinal fluid (CSF), indicative of a skull fracture. The athlete may notice a sweet taste or postnasal drip, which can also be indicative of a CSF leak. Bleeding present in these locations should be assessed by dabbing on tissue paper, which shows a clear ring of wet tissue beyond the blood stain, called a halo or ring sign, when there is also CSF. Analyzing the glucose or tau-transferrin levels can ultimately confirm fluid is CSF. Consideration for CSF leak is important because of the risk for meningitis.[61]

The skull is particularly prone to fracture at certain sites including the temporal and parietal bones, the sphenoid sinus and wings at the skull base, and the foramen magnum. Basilar skull fracture should be suspected in an athlete with battle sign bruising around the mastoid process or raccoon eyes periorbital ecchymosis.

CT scan imaging is the best initial test, often accomplished in the emergency department. Skull fractures are often associated with epidural hematoma.[15]

INTRACRANIAL HEMORRHAGE

Intracranial hemorrhage is the leading cause of death from sports-related head injury.[15]

Categorization includes epidural, subdural, intracerebral, and subarachnoid hemorrhage.

Epidural Hematoma

Damage to the middle meningeal artery, where blood accumulates between the skull and the dura, is often associated with a temporal skull fracture. Epidural hematomas usually result from a high-energy impact (eg, being hit by a baseball). Clinically, there is often a lucid period when the athlete appears to have recovered from initially being stunned or unconscious. The athlete then develops a severe headache and experiences progressive decline in consciousness minutes to hours after the injury. Clot accumulation increases intracranial pressure; hence only neurosurgical expertise can prevent death (with expedient evacuation of a clot, the brain is usually uninjured) **(Fig. 6)**.[14]

Subdural Hematoma

Subdural hematomas are more common than epidural hematomas. Again a high-energy impact that damages the veins beneath the dura mater is responsible. It can

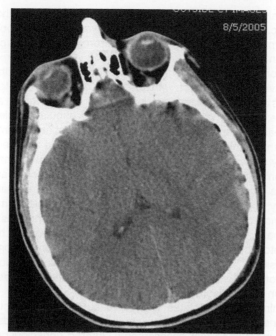

Fig. 6. Epidural hematoma identified on a CT scan of the head. White at the lateral aspect of left hemisphere adjacent to the temporal bone signifies bleeding.

evolve rapidly if there is also a skull fracture. There is a 30% to 40% mortality rate and often residual morbidity if the athlete survives.

Intracerebral Hematoma

This represents bleeding into the brain itself, usually from a torn artery, and it is associated with a very high acceleration injury or congenital abnormality. It is rapidly fatal.

Subarachnoid Hematoma

A subarachnoid hemorrhage is from tearing of the tiny surface brain vessels with bleeding confined to the CSF. It will usually cause headaches and can result in a neurologic deficit, depending on where in the brain is affected, and it often results in seizures. Subarachnoid hematomas can also be rapidly fatal.

INTRACRANIAL INJURY: DIFFUSE AXONAL INJURY

Diffuse axonal injuries are uncommon in sports, because they require severe trauma, resulting in shearing forces that disrupt axonal connections.[18,62] No hematoma is seen on a CT scan. Clinically there is a deep coma, and usually a chronic neurologic deficit, or persistent vegetative state results.

FUNCTIONAL INTRACRANIAL INJURY: CONCUSSION

Concussion is a frequent injury in sports, with skiing, equestrian, and rugby being some of the highest incidence activities worldwide, and football having the highest incidence in the United States.[63–65]

Concussion is also termed mild traumatic brain injury by some authorities; however, suffering a concussion is perhaps the most widely understood. International consensus statements involving expert opinion from around the world have helped define concussion (**Box 1**).[66–68]

Sustaining a concussion requires the brain to be accelerated either in a linear or angular manner via direct contact with the head or indirect contact with another body part such as during a whiplash neck injury.[71] Thresholds for the amount of acceleration are elusive; however, greater than 5000 rad/s/s angular acceleration or greater than 100G of linear acceleration certainly put an athlete at significant risk.[72]

Having experienced this acceleration, the brain is altered at a cellular level rather than showing any evidence of structural injury. Excitatory neurotransmitter activity is thought to predominate, and a period of loss of cerebral vascular autonomy occurs also to create a mismatch of increased brain metabolic demand and relative decreased supply of glucose.[73] These changes may last weeks to months.[74]

During this period of metabolic mismatch, concussion symptoms are manifested. Headache, dizziness, and balance issues are the most common[75]; however, there is a myriad of symptom complexes that can be attributed to concussion and may reflect genetic predisposition,[76] nature of the inciting event, including location of contact and previous history of concussive injury, or other comorbidities such as migraine headaches or attention deficit disorder.

Physical examinations of athletes who have sustained a concussion are often normal beyond the first few minutes from the injury; hence the fieldside examination can be 1 of the most important assessments. Altered consciousness may or may not be present; diplopia or nystagmus can sometimes be elicited. Cerebellar signs such as dysdiadochokinesis can be performed slowly and deliberately, and the ability to balance in a tandem stance with hand on hips and eyes closed is very often diminished with a time of less than 15 seconds without error considered abnormal. Assessment of cognitive function at the fieldside using the SCAT II (Zurich consensus) helps quantify identifiable orientation, memory deficits, and concentration.[68]

With appropriate symptoms or signs of injury, a concussion can be assumed to have occurred. Often there may be a need to exclude a more serious injury such as a skull fracture or intracranial hematoma, necessitating imaging and transfer to an emergency room. However, initial CT or magnetic resonance imaging (MRI) is usually normal in athletes who have sustained a concussion. Once diagnosed as a concussion, acute management will include a period of observation and serial examination. Any deterioration in mental status is not consistent with concussion and should prompt neurosurgical assessment. Concussion symptomatology may worsen the day after an injury, often provoking repeat evaluation. Monitoring of an athlete by a responsible adult in the first 24 to 48 hours after a concussion is essential.

With appropriate cognitive and physical rest, most collegiate athletes who have sustained a concussion will begin to improve over 7 to 10 days.[75] Younger athletes often

---

Box 1
Definition of concussion

"...a complex pathophysiological process affecting the brain, induced by traumatic biomechanical forces..."
International Consensus Statements Sports Concussion[66,69,70]

take longer. The severity of the concussion cannot be predicted, and can only truly be determined retrospectively once the time when all symptoms have resolved has been ascertained. Grading scales documenting loss of consciousness and amnesia have fallen out of favor.

Management decisions in the immediate aftermath of a concussion revolve around avoiding triggers that will worsen symptoms by implementing brain rest strategies such as limiting screen time (eg, television, cell phone, computer, video games) and physical activity. Decisions about timing of return to school often must be individualized and should be determined by a physician. Once symptoms have completely resolved, a return to physical activity can be attempted. This is best accomplished with a progressive, stepwise return to sport (e.g. aerobic exercise, strength and conditioning, skills practice, contact practice, scrimmage, competitive play). If symptoms recur with any step, the athlete should revert to the previous level for 1 to 2 days and not progress further until symptoms have again resolved. This progression takes at least 5 to 7 days to achieve a return to competitive contact sport when each step is tolerated without increased symptoms.

Cumulative injury from repeat concussions is a very real risk, and this is thought to occur after 3 separate concussions.[77,78] The possibility of ultimately sustaining chronic traumatic encephalopathy later in life is an alarming newly identified risk, with years of contact sport and repetitive concussion events probably responsible.

A failure to avoid further head trauma while recovering from an original concussive injury can have severe, and rarely life-threatening, consequences. Second-impact syndrome has been described as a period of susceptibility to accelerated cerebral edema, coma, and death due to brainstem herniation, which is thought to happen after a second impact to the head while still symptomatic and recovering from the first impact.

Determining recovery after a concussion should include resolution of symptoms and normalization of physical examination. This can be supplemented with neuropsychological testing or balance testing, both of which have been validated in use in sports concussion.[79–82]

Best practices in prevention of concussion involves preparticipation examinations to elicit history of previous head injuries, consideration of baseline neuropsychological or balance testing, and education of all involved in the care of an athlete or team to the risk of concussion and the difficulties in identifying this often subtle condition. Equipment has not been shown to prevent concussion to date, and helmets are worn to prevent structural injury rather than functional brain injury.[83] Some studies have shown increased incidence of injury in sports such as rugby with the use of headgear.[84]

SUMMARY

Closed-head injuries vary from the very minor to the catastrophic. It is often difficult to differentiate the severity at initial presentation. Serial assessment is very valuable, and cannot be understated in terms of value in excluding serious intracranial injury. Awareness of facial injuries is aided by familiarity with facial bone anatomy and the clinical presentation of orbital, zygomatic, maxillary, and mandibular fracture. Functional injury such as concussion may coexist with other injuries and requires a careful evaluation, which should include a sideline assessment tool, and may include balance and neuropsychological tracking of recovery. Helmets may not always protect against intracranial injury.

REFERENCES

1. Kelly KD, Lissel HL, Rowe BH, et al. Sport and recreation-related head injuries treated in the emergency department. Clin J Sport Med 2001;11(2):77–81.
2. Kerr HA, Curtis C, Micheli LJ, et al. Collegiate rugby union injury patterns in New England: a prospective cohort study. Br J Sports Med 2008;42(7):595–603.
3. Kemp SP, Hudson Z, Brooks JH, et al. The epidemiology of head injuries in English professional rugby union. Clin J Sport Med 2008;18(3):227–34.
4. Niedfeldt MW. Head injuries, heading, and the use of headgear in soccer. Curr Sports Med Rep 2011;10(6):324–9.
5. Boden BP, Kirkendall DT, Garrett WE Jr. Concussion incidence in elite college soccer players. Am J Sports Med 1998;26(2):238–41.
6. Chaze B, McDonald P. Head injuries in winter sports: downhill skiing, snowboarding, sledding, snowmobiling, ice skating and ice hockey. Neurol Clin 2008;26(1):325–32, xii–xiii.
7. McIntosh AS, Andersen TE, Bahr R, et al. Sports helmets now and in the future. Br J Sports Med 2011;45(16):1258–65.
8. Benson BW, Hamilton GM, Meeuwisse WH, et al. Is protective equipment useful in preventing concussion? A systematic review of the literature. Br J Sports Med 2009;43(Suppl 1):i56–67.
9. Benson BW, Rose MS, Meeuwisse WH. The impact of face shield use on concussions in ice hockey: a multivariate analysis. Br J Sports Med 2002;36(1): 27–32.
10. Vinger PF. Eye injury resulting from violence. Research and prevention. Arch Ophthalmol 1992;110(6):765–6.
11. Ferrari LR. The injured eye. Anesthesiol Clin North America 1996;14(1):125–50.
12. Pizzarello LD, Haik BG. Sports ophthalmology. Springfield (IL): Charles C. Thomas Books; 1987.
13. Rodriguez JO, Lavina AM, Agarwal A. Prevention and treatment of common eye injuries in sports. Am Fam Physician 2003;67(7):1481–8.
14. Purcell L. Traumatic head injury. In: Micheli L, Purcell L, editors. The adolescent athlete: a practical approach. New York: Springer; 2007. p. 61–79.
15. Proctor MR, Cantu RC. Head and neck injuries in young athletes. Clin Sports Med 2000;19(4):693–715.
16. Cantu RC, Bailes JE, Wilberger JE Jr. Guidelines for return to contact or collision sport after a cervical spine injury. Clin Sports Med 1998;17(1):137–46.
17. Smith BW. Head injuries. In: Harris S, Anderson S, editors. Care of the young athlete. 2nd edition. Elk Grove Village, (IL): American Academy of Pediatrics; 2009. p. 171.
18. Warren WL Jr, Bailes JE. On the field evaluation of athletic head injuries. Clin Sports Med 1998;17(1):13–26.
19. Warren WL Jr, Bailes JE. On the field evaluation of athletic neck injury. Clin Sports Med 1998;17(1):99–110.
20. Maddocks DL, Dicker GD, Saling MM. The assessment of orientation following concussion in athletes. Clin J Sport Med 1995;5(1):32–5.
21. Jinguji TM, Bompadre V, Harmon KG, et al. Sport Concussion Assessment Tool 2: baseline values for high school athletes. Br J Sports Med 2012;46(5):365–70.
22. Schneider KJ, Emery CA, Kang J, et al. Examining Sport Concussion Assessment Tool ratings for male and female youth hockey players with and without a history of concussion. Br J Sports Med 2010;44(15):1112–7.
23. Teasdale G. Assessment of head injuries. Br J Anaesth 1976;48(8):761–6.

24. Hunte G. Sporting emergencies. In: Brukner P, Khan K, editors. Clinical sports medicine. 2nd edition. Roseville, New South Wales, Australia: McGraw-Hill; 2001. p. 713–25.
25. Toriumi DM, Lovice D, O'Grady KM. Fibrin tissue adhesive in otolaryngology-head and neck surgery. J Long Term Eff Med Implants 1998;8(2):143–59.
26. Trott AT. Wounds and Lacerations: Emergency Care and Closure. In: Marx J, Hockberger R, Walls R, editors. In Rosen's Emergency Medicine-Concepts and Clinical Practice. Philadelphia, PA: Elsevier, mosby; 2005.
27. Shumrick KA, Chadwell JB. Facial trauma: soft-tissue lacerations and burns. 4th edition. Philadelphia: Mosby; 2005.
28. Macdonald DJ, Calder N, Perrett G, et al. Case presentation: a novel way of treating acute cauliflower ear in a professional rugby player. Br J Sports Med 2005; 39(6):e29.
29. Choung YH, Park K, Choung PH, et al. Simple compressive method for treatment of auricular haematoma using dental silicone material. J Laryngol Otol 2005; 119(1):27–31.
30. George A, Tassone P. Pinna haematomas of the conchal bowl. Clin Otolaryngol 2007;32(1):77.
31. Wilson BD. Protective headgear in rugby union. Sports Med 1998;25(5):333–7.
32. Reehal P. Facial injury in sport. Curr Sports Med Rep 2010;9(1):27–34.
33. Stewart MG. Head, face, and neck trauma: comprehensive management. New York: Thieme; 2005.
34. Perry M, Dancey A, Mireskandari K, et al. Emergency care in facial trauma—a maxillofacial and ophthalmic perspective. Injury 2005;36(8):875–96.
35. Bord SP, Linden J. Trauma to the globe and orbit. Emerg Med Clin North Am 2008;26(1):97–123, vi–vii.
36. Hislop WS, Dutton GN, Douglas PS. Treatment of retrobulbar haemorrhage in accident and emergency departments. Br J Oral Maxillofac Surg 1996;34(4):289–92.
37. Flores MT, Andersson L, Andreasen JO, et al. Guidelines for the management of traumatic dental injuries. II. Avulsion of permanent teeth. Dent Traumatol 2007; 23(3):130–6.
38. Flores MT, Andersson L, Andreasen JO, et al. Guidelines for the management of traumatic dental injuries. I. Fractures and luxations of permanent teeth. Dent Traumatol 2007;23(2):66–71.
39. Flores MT, Malmgren B, Andersson L, et al. Guidelines for the management of traumatic dental injuries. III. Primary teeth. Dent Traumatol 2007;23(4):196–202.
40. Kerr IL, Bigsby GA, Haeseler GA. Prevention and emergency first-aid treatment for sports-related dentofacial injuries. Compendium 1993;14(9):1142, 1144–6 passim; quiz: 56.
41. Howe AS. Craniomaxillofacial injuries. In: Seidenberg PH, Beutler AI, editors. The sports medicine resource manual. Philadelphia: Saunders Elsevier; 2008. p. 253–71.
42. Ranalli DN. Dental injuries in sports. Curr Sports Med Rep 2005;4(1):12–7.
43. Mourouzis C, Koumoura F. Sports-related maxillofacial fractures: a retrospective study of 125 patients. Int J Oral Maxillofac Surg 2005;34(6):635–8.
44. Bayliss T, Bedi R. Oral, maxillofacial, and general injuries in gymnasts. Injury 1996;27(5):353–4.
45. Carroll SM, Jawad MA, West M, et al. One hundred and ten sports-related facial fractures. Br J Sports Med 1995;29(3):194–5.
46. Kellman RM. Maxillofacial trauma. In: Cummings CW, Flint PW, Robbins KT, editors. Otolaryngology: head & neck surgery. 4th edition. Philadelphia: Mosby; 2005;23:318–41.

47. Petrigliano FA, Williams RJ 3rd. Orbital fractures in sport: a review. Sports Med 2003;33(4):317–22.
48. Brady SM, McMann MA, RA M. The diagnosis and management of orbital blowout fractures: update 2001. Am J Emerg Med 2001;19:148–54.
49. Cappuccino GJ, Rhee ST, MS G. Maxillofacial injuries. In: Asensio JA, Trunkey DD, editors. Current therapy of trauma and surgical critical care. 1st edition. Philadelphia (PA): Mosby Elsevier; 2008;27:175–81.
50. Kelley P, Hopper R, Gruss J. Evaluation and treatment of zygomatic fractures. Plast Reconstr Surg 2007;120(7 Suppl 2):5S–15S.
51. Fraioli RE, Branstetter BF, Deleyiannis FW. Facial fractures: beyond Le Fort. Otolaryngol Clin North Am 2008;41(1):51–76, vi.
52. Manson PN, Hoopes JE, Su CT. Structural pillars of the facial skeleton: an approach to the management of Le Fort fractures. Plast Reconstr Surg 1980; 66(1):54–62.
53. Burton JH, Armellino N. Facial trauma. In: Adams JG, Barton ED, Collings J, et al, editors. Emergency Medicine. Philadelphia (PA): Saunders; 2008;71:661–72.
54. Higuera S, Lee EI, Cole P, et al. Nasal trauma and the deviated nose. Plast Reconstr Surg 2007;120(7 Suppl 2):64S–75S.
55. Kucik CJ, Clenney T, Phelan J. Management of acute nasal fractures. Am Fam Physician 2004;70(7):1315–20.
56. Rohrich RJ, Adams WP Jr. Nasal fracture management: minimizing secondary nasal deformities. Plast Reconstr Surg 2000;106(2):266–73.
57. Seshul MB, Sinn DP, Gerlock AJ Jr. The Andy Gump fracture of the mandible: a cause of respiratory obstruction or distress. J Trauma 1978;18(8):611–2.
58. Bavitz JB, Collicott PE. Bilateral mandibular subcondylar fractures contributing to airway obstruction. Int J Oral Maxillofac Surg 1995;24(4):273–5.
59. Roccia F, Bianchi F, Zavattero E, et al. Characteristics of maxillofacial trauma in females: a retrospective analysis of 367 patients. J Craniomaxillofac Surg 2010; 38(4):314–9.
60. Putukian M, Harmon KG. Head injuries. In: Birrer R, Griesemer B, Cataletto M, editors. Pediatric sports medicine for primary care. Philadelphia: Lippincott, Williams & Wilkins; 2002. p. 266–90.
61. Rice DH. Management of frontal sinus fractures. Curr Opin Otolaryngol Head Neck Surg 2004;12(1):46–8.
62. Cantu RC. Return to play guidelines after a head injury. Clin Sports Med 1998; 17(1):45–60.
63. McIntosh AS, McCrory P. Preventing head and neck injury. Br J Sports Med 2005; 39(6):314–8.
64. Koh JO, Cassidy JD, Watkinson EJ. Incidence of concussion in contact sports: a systematic review of the evidence. Brain Inj 2003;17(10):901–17.
65. Grindel SH. Epidemiology and pathophysiology of minor traumatic brain injury. Curr Sports Med Rep 2003;2(1):18–23.
66. Aubry M, Cantu R, Dvorak J, et al. Summary and agreement statement of the 1st International Symposium on Concussion in Sport, Vienna 2001. Clin J Sport Med 2002;12(1):6–11.
67. Fuller CW, Molloy MG, Bagate C, et al. Consensus statement on injury definitions and data collection procedures for studies of injuries in rugby union. Clin J Sport Med 2007;17(3):177–81.
68. McCrory P, Meeuwisse W, Johnston K, et al. Consensus statement on concussion in sport—the Third International Conference on Concussion in Sport held in Zurich, November 2008. Phys Sportsmed 2009;37(2):141–59.

69. McCrory P, Johnston K, Meeuwisse W, et al. Summary and agreement statement of the 2nd International Conference on Concussion in Sport, Prague 2004. Br J Sports Med 2005;39(4):196–204.

70. McCrory P, Meeuwisse W, Johnston K, et al. Consensus statement on concussion in sport—the 3rd International Conference on concussion in sport, held in Zurich, November 2008. J Clin Neurosci 2009;16(6):755–63.

71. Barth JT, Freeman JR, Broshek DK, et al. Acceleration-deceleration sport-related concussion: the gravity of it all. J Athl Train 2001;36(3):253–6.

72. Guskiewicz KM, Mihalik JP. Biomechanics of sport concussion: quest for the elusive injury threshold. Exerc Sport Sci Rev 2011;39(1):4–11.

73. Gennarelli TA, Graham DI. Neuropathology of the head injuries. Semin Clin Neuropsychiatry 1998;3(3):160–75.

74. Giza CC, Hovda DA. The neurometabolic cascade of concussion. J Athl Train 2001;36(3):228–35.

75. Guskiewicz KM, McCrea M, Marshall SW, et al. Cumulative effects associated with recurrent concussion in collegiate football players: the NCAA Concussion Study. JAMA 2003;290(19):2549–55.

76. Blackman JA, Worley G, Strittmatter WJ. Apolipoprotein E and brain injury: implications for children. Dev Med Child Neurol 2005;47(1):64–70.

77. Meehan WP 3rd, Bachur RG. Sport-related concussion. Pediatrics 2009;123(1): 114–23.

78. Iverson GL, Gaetz M, Lovell MR, et al. Cumulative effects of concussion in amateur athletes. Brain Inj 2004;18(5):433–43.

79. Iverson GL, Lovell MR, Collins MW. Interpreting change on ImPACT following sport concussion. Clin Neuropsychol 2003;17(4):460–7.

80. Collins MW, Grindel SH, Lovell MR, et al. Relationship between concussion and neuropsychological performance in college football players. JAMA 1999;282(10): 964–70.

81. Grindel SH, Lovell MR, Collins MW. The assessment of sport-related concussion: the evidence behind neuropsychological testing and management. Clin J Sport Med 2001;11(3):134–43.

82. Guskiewicz KM. Balance assessment in the management of sport-related concussion. Clin Sports Med 2011;30(1):89–102, ix.

83. Guskiewicz KM, Bruce SL, Cantu RC, et al. National Athletic Trainers' Association position statement: management of sport-related concussion. J Athl Train 2004; 39(3):280–97.

84. Hollis SJ, Stevenson MR, McIntosh AS, et al. Mild traumatic brain injury among a cohort of rugby union players: predictors of time to injury. Br J Sports Med 2011;45(12):997–9.

Blunt Visual Trauma

Giselle A. Aerni, MD[a,b,*]

KEYWORDS

- Visual trauma • Protective eyewear • Corneal abrasion • Orbital blowout fracture

KEY POINTS

- The incidence of eye injuries from sporting events has ranged from 4.1% to 13.7%, reported in the literature.
- Recommendations for protective eyewear vary by sport and should be considered as part of an overall injury prevention plan.
- Corneal abrasions are evaluated with fluorescein staining, treated with cycloplegics and antibiotics, and should resolve within 3 days.
- A hyphema is blood in the anterior chamber and represents an injury that should be referred to ophthalmology immediately because of the risk of severe complications.
- The classic symptom in an orbital blowout fracture is double vision with vertical gaze.

Blunt visual trauma injuries are common in sports and can encompass a wide range of severity. The sports medicine physician must be able to identify and manage a variety of injuries. Consideration should be given to the use of protective eyewear, especially in the case of the functionally one-eyed athlete.

This article reviews visual trauma injury patterns in different sports, evidence and controversy surrounding protective eyewear, and some common clinical entities that are seen with blunt visual trauma.

INCIDENCE

Ocular trauma in athletes can have devastating consequences. Incidence of eye injuries from sporting events has ranged over the years from 4.1% to 13.7%.[1–3] These injuries may be minor, such as a periorbital contusion, but can also involve severe injuries, such as hyphema and globe rupture. Different sports have different inherent risks, and some require eye protection equipment for competition, also altering their risk patterns.

Funding Sources: None.
Conflict of Interest: None.
[a] 263 Farmington Avenue, Mail Code 7140, Farmington, CT 06032, USA; [b] Department of Sports Medicine, University of Connecticut, 505 Stadium Road, Unit 3204, Storrs, CT 06269, USA
* Family Medicine Center at Asylum Hill, 99 Woodland Street, Hartford, CT 06105, USA.
E-mail address: gaerni@stfranciscare.org

Each year in the United States more than 40,000 eye injuries occur from sports.[4] Sports with small, hard, fast projectiles and sticks have the highest risk of injury, including rifle, paintball, squash, lacrosse, and racquetball. Additionally, boxing and contact martial arts have a very high risk. Soccer, water polo, and football have a moderate risk, and swimming and bicycling have a low risk.

A decade-long retrospective study from 1988 to 1999 in Norway showed that 13.7% of eye injuries presenting to the ophthalmology department were associated with a sport.[1] The mechanism of injury was most often from a ball (71.1%) or a club (13.2%). They reported that the highest incidence was noted in soccer (35.5%). A similar study performed in Scotland showed that 12.5% of ocular injuries admitted to the hospital were sport-related.[2] This study also found that soccer had the highest number of injuries at 32.5% but that all racquet sports combined accounted for 47.5% of injuries. Capao Filipe and colleagues[3] reviewed sports-related eye injuries and found that 8.3% of injuries presenting to an eye emergency department were caused by modern sports, such as paintball and motocross. These studies were all performed in high-acuity settings, inpatient settings, and emergency departments. Thus, they likely underestimate the full scope of injuries that occur and never reach such a level of care.

SPORT-SPECIFIC INJURIES

The incidence and risk pattern of blunt visual trauma can vary based on the different sporting events. Type of play, rules of the game, and protective eyewear requirements can all change the numbers and types of injuries seen. A few examples are listed herein.

Soccer

It is interesting that soccer should have one of the highest incidences of ocular injury, because the ball is very large compared with the diameter of the orbit. Capao Felipe[5] describes the unique mechanism of injury caused by the soccer ball itself: "orbital penetration is lower, but the time in the orbit is longer and, during rebound, a secondary suction effect is produced on the orbital contents." In a separate study, Capao Felipe and colleagues[6] found that the most common initial diagnosis of an eye injury in soccer was eyelid or orbital contusion and hyphema, followed by retinal hemorrhage, vitreous hemorrhage, and uveitis. At follow-up, the most frequent diagnosis was angle recession and retinal tears. This finding suggests that some injuries may either be missed at initial diagnosis or have a delayed presentation. With any severe visual trauma, follow-up is important.

Boxing

Ophthalmologic examination of 956 Italian Boxing Federation boxers was compared with 80 male controls to evaluate the prevalence and nature of ocular injuries in boxers over almost 2 decades, from 1982 to 1998.[7] The boxers did have a higher prevalence of milder ocular injury (40.9%) compared with controls (3.1%); however, they did not have a significantly higher prevalence of severe lesions compared with controls (5.6% vs 3.1%). Other studies have shown that a higher percentage of boxers actually do have pronounced or vision-threatening ocular injuries, as high as 21% to 58%.[8]

Giovinazzo and colleagues[8] found a linear correlation between number of fights lost and the incidence of retinal tears. The probability of retinal tear additionally increased with the number of bouts, showing a 90% probability after 75 bouts. Previously, thumbing injuries such as optic nerve avulsion, carried a greater concern. However, with the advent of thumbless gloves, the incidence of thumbing injuries has decreased.[9]

Golf

Although golf does not contribute a large overall number of ocular injuries to sport-related eye trauma, it does have a significantly higher proportion of severe or catastrophic injuries. Weitgasser and colleagues[10] performed a retrospective study from 1993 to 2000 and identified only 7 golf-related eye injuries: 6 were from the golf ball and 1 from a club. Of the patients, 4 had an open globe injury, 2 required orbital floor fracture surgery, and 3 enucleations had to be performed. In a review of pediatric patients, 11 total injuries occurred over a 15-year period: 10 injuries from the club and 1 from a ball.[11] These severe injuries included orbital fracture, hyphema, and traumatic optic neuropathy. Of these children, 9 required surgical intervention and 3 had permanent deficits, including blindness, decreased vision, and anophthalmia.

PREPARTICIPATION EXAMINATION

The *PPE Preparticipation Physical Evaluation, 4th Edition*, asks 4 historical questions regarding the eyes:

1. Have you had any problems with your eyes or vision?
2. Have you had any eye injuries?
3. Do you wear glasses or contact lenses?
4. Do you wear protective eyewear, such as goggles or a face shield?

The physical examination consists of checking visual acuity and evaluating for equal pupils.[12]

The American Academy of Pediatrics (AAP) and the American Academy of Ophthalmology (AAO) issued a joint statement in 2004 recommending that athletes who are functionally one-eyed wear protective eyewear during all sports and should not participate in boxing or full-contact martial arts.[13] A functionally one-eyed athlete has a best-corrected visual acuity of worse than 20/40 in the poorer-seeing eye. The concern is that if the better eye becomes injured, the athlete may essentially lose all vision or become severely limited in sight.

PROTECTIVE EYEWEAR

There is much debate across different sports regarding the use and benefit of protective eyewear. The AAP and AAO joint statement on protective eyewear recommends that all youths involved in sports be encouraged to wear appropriate eye protection, and provides a list of recommended eye protectors for specific sports.[13] They additionally stress that contact lenses do not protect the eye or vision and that athletes who wear contacts also need to wear protective eyewear.

Squash carries a high risk of eye injuries and has a fair amount of literature regarding the use of protective eyewear and general attitudes toward eye protection. A survey of Australian squash players, performed in 1989, 1995, and 2000, showed an increase over time in the self-reported use of eyewear; however, only half of the players who used eye protection used appropriate eyewear.[14] Attitudes toward eye protection also improved over time, with an increasing number of players feeling that squash players should use some type of eyewear and that eye protection should be mandatory for juniors. When reviewing beliefs and attitudes of venue operators, some did believe that more players should use protective eyewear; however, most believed that players with more experience did not need the protection.[15] Additionally, very few venues had eyewear available for borrow or purchase. A protective eyewear promotion strategy was shown to be effective in increasing the odds that a player would wear appropriate eyewear.[16]

Attitudes toward protective eyewear are improving, and work is being done to test equipment. Baker and colleagues[17] performed a study to evaluate the optical and impact performance of football protective faceshields. They were able to show that the faceshields did not fracture, even with impact velocities up to 66.4 m/s, and had good optical quality. However, the study was not designed to evaluate for a possible decreased risk of eye injury in a sport in which almost 20% of injuries are caused by fingers penetrating helmets to the eyes. In soccer, data exist showing that protective eyewear that complies with standard ASTM F803 can prevent contact of the ball to the eye.[18]

As rules requiring the use of protective eyewear in sports are being mandated, outcomes data regarding injury-prevention efficacy are following behind. Retrospective data from Australian women's lacrosse, in which eye gear is not mandatory, indicate that eye injuries account for 12.2% of all injuries to the head.[19] In the United States, US Lacrosse mandated the use of protective eyewear in women's lacrosse during the 2004–2005 season. Lincoln and colleagues performed a cohort study comparing eye injury rates before and after implementation of the protective eyewear mandate and found that the rate of eye injuries decreased from 0.10 to 0.016 injuries per 1000 athlete exposures.[20]

In the sport of hurling, outcomes data show a significant reduction in eye injuries after sporting rules were changed requiring protective head gear and face masks for all players aged 18 years and younger.[21] In the sport of ice hockey, National Hockey League players who wear a facemask have a significantly decreased risk of eye injury compared with those who choose not to use a facemask.[22]

Although outcomes data are still fairly limited, those that have been collected seem to show a benefit to using protective eyewear in sports.

BLUNT TRAUMA INJURIES

Overall, sports carry an increased risk of eye injury that the sports medicine physician must be aware of and able to manage appropriately. Following are specific examples of blunt trauma injuries and their management.

Periorbital Contusion

Periorbital contusion can occur in athletes participating in contact and ball sports, and unfortunately can also be seen in individuals as a result of outside activities (**Fig. 1**).

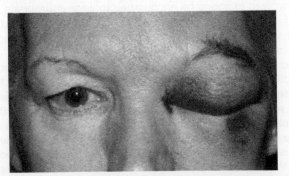

Fig. 1. Periorbital contusion. (*From* Boruchoff SA. Anterior segment disease: a diagnostic color atlas. Philadelphia: Elsiever; 2001. p. 204; with permission.)

A contusion typically looks worse than it is and involves ecchymosis and edema of the periorbital tissues that can track to the contralateral eye.

A thorough examination should be performed to rule out any fracture or injury to the globe, and if no concomitant injury is seen, treatment with a cold compress is all that is required. Athletes with substantial bruising and swelling should undergo nonemergent follow-up with an ophthalmologist for a full retinal evaluation, because the trauma can cause slight tears in the retinal periphery, which are not initially symptomatic but can cause delayed retinal detachment.

Eyelid Trauma and Laceration

In the event of eyelid trauma, avulsion, or laceration, the goal of the sports medicine physician is to evaluate for other injuries to the globe and facilitate referral to an ophthalmologist (**Fig. 2**).

Isolated lid injuries are repaired with consideration of corneal exposure and cosmetic appearance. Complications can include incomplete closure of the eyelids, corneal irritation from misdirected eyelashes, canalicular injuries, and retrobulbar hemorrhage. Generally the prognosis is very good with timely repair; however, scarring and altered cosmetic appearance can require additional procedures for correction in the future.

Corneal Abrasion

An athlete can sustain a corneal abrasion with even mild trauma to the eye, typically from a finger or fingernail during a game. However, this can also occur outside of competition from contact lens difficulty, makeup brushes, or other foreign bodies.

Athletes will experience pain and a sensation that something is in the eye. They often have photophobia, conjunctival injection, and blepharospasm. Decreased vision will only be seen in a central corneal abrasion (**Fig. 3**).

Occasionally, the surface irregularity caused by the abrasion can be seen with just a penlight; however, the best way to visualize an abrasion is with fluorescein dye. Fluorescein stains areas where the epithelium has been removed and provides a map of the abrasion. Using a topical anesthetic confirms the diagnosis when it provides immediate relief to the patient.

It is important to evert the eyelids to look for any foreign body that may still be present and can cause continued abrasions. Additionally, if no recent trauma has

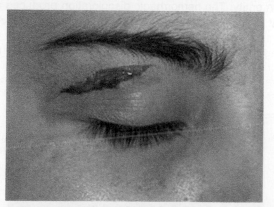

Fig. 2. Eyelid laceration. (*From* Thomsen T, Setnik G, editors. Procedures Consult. Nerve blocks of the face. Copyright 2008 Elsevier Inc. All rights reserved; used with permission. Available at: http://www.proceduresconsult.com/medical-procedures/nerve-blocks-of-the-face-EM-019-procedure.aspx. Accessed Mar 15, 2013.)

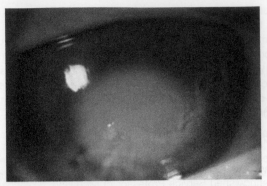

Fig. 3. Corneal abrasion, as visualized with fluorescein staining under blue lamp. (*From* Goldman L, Ausiello D. Cecil text book of medicine, 22nd edition. Philadelphia: WB Saunders; 2004; with permission.)

occurred to cause the abrasion, it is likely that the patient developed a recurrent erosion because of problems with reepithelialization of a past injury.

Treatment of injuries not associated with contact lenses involves using a cycloplegic agent 2 to 3 times a day and an antibiotic ointment 3 times a day. Pressure patching should be avoided unless performed under the guidance of an ophthalmologist because of the increased risk for infection. If the abrasion was associated with contact lens use, the antibiotic chosen must provide coverage for gram-negative organisms (*Pseudomonas*), and must be applied 4 to 6 times a day.

Corneal abrasions should be regularly monitored until resolution. Referral to ophthalmology should be made if healing takes longer than 3 days, if there is a large central abrasion, or if the abrasion is at high-risk for infection. Athletes who wear contact lenses will need to refrain from lens use until the injury is completely healed. If lens use caused the injury, such as in overuse or tight lens syndrome, it should be discontinued until the patient has been evaluated by an ophthalmologist to optimize corneal health.

Subconjunctival Hemorrhage

Although subconjunctival hemorrhage can be disconcerting in appearance, it is actually a fairly benign entity. The hemorrhagic discoloration produces a bright red area that may be fairly focal or more diffuse in the anterior sclera (**Fig. 4**). It is often first

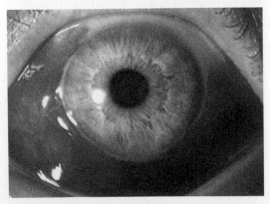

Fig. 4. Subconjunctival hemorrhage. (*From* Wirbelauer C. Management of the red eye for the primary care physician. Am J Med 2006;119(4):302–6; with permission.)

noticed on awakening and can be caused by minor trauma or a Valsalva maneuver (eg, coughing, heavy lifting).

With a benign cause, such as minimal trauma or a Valsalva history, the patient can be reassured, provided with artificial tears as needed, and told to expect the blood to clear in approximately 2 weeks. Even though the hemorrhage can be frightening in appearance to an athlete, the prognosis is excellent.

It is important to keep in mind that some causes of subconjunctival hemorrhage may actually be much more serious. If the hemorrhage was caused by high-velocity projectiles or other severe trauma, the possibility exists that the hemorrhage could be hiding a ruptured globe, and therefore a more thorough evaluation must be performed. Additionally, complete subconjunctival hemorrhage about the entire 360° globe can indicate a more serious abnormality, such as periorbital fracture, retrobulbar hematoma, or bleeding disorder. The history and examination will provide clues as to whether a more serious entity should be considered.

Hyphema

A hyphema is blood in the anterior chamber that is caused by blunt trauma. It is a much more serious red-eye condition that is associated with severe complications (**Fig. 5**).

The athlete will present with a history of blunt trauma followed by pain, blurred vision, and a red eye. Red blood cells can be seen in the anterior chamber in suspension (microhyphema) or layered out. Despite most textbook images showing layering at 6 o'clock, the blood will always layer at the most dependent portion of the patient's anterior chamber, which depends on how the patient has been positioned (eg, sitting, lying down).

It is most important to shield (not patch) the eye and have the athlete evaluated by ophthalmology immediately. The ophthalmologist will evaluate and follow intraocular pressure, and evaluate for any periorbital injuries, intraocular injuries, corneal blood staining, and rebleeding. Treatment involves eye shielding for protection, bed rest with minimal careful ambulation, and cycloplegic agents twice a day. Patients are also often provided with antiemetic medicines and acetaminophen for pain.

Any African American athlete who has not already been screened for sickle cell trait should be screened, because this adds a level of complication in patients with sickle cell trait or disease. Even patients with sickle cell trait can have difficulty clearing red

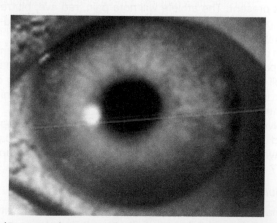

Fig. 5. Hyphema. (*From* Krachmer JH. The red eye. In: Paley DA, Krachmer JH, editors. Primary Care Ophthalmology, 2nd edition. Philadelphia: Mosby, 2005; with permission.)

blood cells from the anterior chamber, causing a significant increase in intraocular pressure 1 to 2 days after the injury. Keeping the pressure at lower levels in these patients is critical to avoid inhibiting optic nerve head perfusion.

In the event of microhyphema and small hyphemas without other injuries, the overall prognosis is fairly good. However, in patients with large hyphemas, rebleeds, and sickle cell disease or trait, the prognosis is more concerning, with long-term complications including glaucoma, permanent corneal staining, and retinal injury.

Foreign Body

Although intraocular foreign body injuries do not typically occur as the result of blunt trauma, failure to recognize an intraocular foreign body can result in vision loss, and thus must always be considered in the differential of visual trauma.

Patients may have pain, red eye, and photophobia, with varied decreases in vision. Typically they have a history suggestive of penetrating injury. These patients must all be referred to ophthalmology.

Foreign bodies can also lodge themselves within the conjunctiva and cornea. Superficial material can be removed by the sports medicine physician, whereas any injuries that are suspected or seen to extend deeply must be referred to ophthalmology for safe evaluation, treatment, and management.

Scleral Laceration or Globe Rupture

Scleral laceration or rupture is a severe ophthalmologic emergency. Laceration typically involves trauma with a high-speed projectile or sharp object and is only rarely partial thickness. Scleral injury that results in complete globe rupture is often caused by severe blunt trauma from a fist, club, or ball.

The athlete will have a history of trauma and present with red eye, pain, decreased vision, and possible blepharospasm. A defect may be seen; however, significant swelling or hemorrhagic suffusion may hide a scleral injury. If a scleral injury or rupture is seen or suspected, the eye must be protected with a shield (taking care to minimize any manipulation of the globe) and the patient referred to ophthalmology immediately for evaluation and possible surgical repair.

Traumatic Iritis

In cases of traumatic iritis, the blunt traumatic event has typically occurred 2 to 3 days before symptoms present. The athlete will note pain, red eye, blurred vision, photophobia, and tearing. Iritis occurs because of a breakdown in the blood-aqueous barrier caused by intraocular inflammation.

On examination conjunctival injection with a ciliary flush will be seen. The patient will have consensual pain in the affected eye when light is directed into the uninvolved eye. The affected pupil may appear sluggish to react, and may also be constricted. The anterior chamber will demonstrate cell and flare pattern. With significant trauma, it is important to check intraocular pressure.

Treatment involves cycloplegic agents 3 times a day. Ophthalmology may choose to use corticosteroid drops as long as no infection is present and the patient has appropriate follow-up available. The athlete should undergo close follow-up and can expect resolution within 7 to 10 days.

Traumatic Retrobulbar Hemorrhage

When blunt trauma to the orbit occurs, arteries within the orbital cavity can be injured, causing an increase in intraorbital pressure that results in anterior displacement of the globe. As the globe is pressed forward, the resistance from anterior bony and soft tissue structures causes an increase in intraocular pressure, which can eventually lead to optic nerve damage and central retinal artery compromise.

The athlete will present with pain, decreased vision, and marked swelling. As the blood tracks along tissue planes, the patient may develop a massive subconjunctival hemorrhage whose posterior borders cannot be visualized. The forward pressure causes proptosis and on palpation a tense orbit is noted by significant resistance on retropulsion of the globe. The patient will frequently have limited extraocular movements. Pupil reactions should be normal; however, if a relative afferent pupillary defect develops, it is an indication of optic nerve injury, either from the compression itself or a traumatic optic neuropathy (see later discussion).

It is important to evaluate the fundus and assess intraocular pressure; however, with significant retrobulbar hemorrhage, the patient should be referred to ophthalmology. Treatment can involve medication to decrease intraocular pressure, but may need to advance to surgery to decrease pressure via eyelid surgery or anterior chamber tap. These patients require daily follow-up with careful monitoring of their intraocular pressure.

Orbital Blowout Fracture

One-third of orbital blowout fractures occur during sports participation.[23] Orbital blowout fractures may be caused by significant blunt trauma to the orbital rim, causing direct fracture extending into the floor of the orbit, or by compression of the soft tissues of the orbit, causing indirect fracture internally from forces that push out against very thin orbital walls. Most injuries are to the orbital floor (**Fig. 6**).

Pain can be variable in athletes with a blowout fracture, and the classical symptom is double vision with vertical gaze. If the athlete notes swelling of the eyelids after sneezing or blowing the nose, this indicates a communication between the sinuses and the orbit. The athlete may have enophthalmos, restricted extraocular movements, and tenderness to palpation of the orbital rim.

The patient should be evaluated for injury to the globe itself as well as for any air entrapment (orbital emphysema) within the orbit. Cheek sensation should be assessed to evaluate for injury to the infraorbital nerve.

This injury requires referral to ophthalmology for a complete examination, which should also be repeated 1 week after the injury as the initial edema resolves.

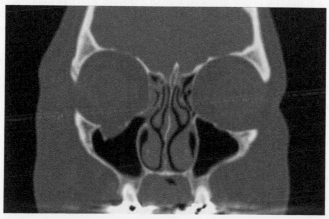

Fig. 6. Coronal CT image showing fracture to the orbital floor of the right orbit.

Treatment involves nasal decongestants and antibiotics if concern exists regarding sinus disease or a communication between the sinuses and the orbit. Additionally, cold compresses are used to reduce edema. Athletes must be advised to avoid blowing their nose and sneezing, if possible.

Some athletes may require surgical repair of the orbital floor in the presence of persistent entrapment, gross enophthalmos, diminished extraocular muscle mobility, and extremely large fractures.

Patients must be monitored for fevers, increasing pain, and erythema, because these may be signs of a developing cellulitis.

Traumatic Optic Neuropathy

Optic neuropathy has direct and indirect origins. The optic nerve can undergo direct compression by bone fragments, foreign body, or edema. Additionally, the optic nerve can undergo a shearing injury from blunt trauma to the head.

The athlete will have decreased visual acuity that is not explained by refractive error or injury to the retina, lens, or cornea. The patient may especially have difficulty with color vision and red saturation. In fact, perceived loss of central red recognition in the involved eye is a strong indicator of potential optic nerve injury. The development of a relative afferent pupillary defect should also suggest the diagnosis.

The diagnostic workup should include a complete eye examination, including visual fields, acuity, and color vision testing. CT scan of the orbits and head can show compressive injuries to the nerve not visualized on examination.

Treatment and management of this abnormality are performed by ophthalmology, and typically involve high-dose corticosteroids. If the patient has developed an afferent pupillary defect, the injury to the optic nerve is likely more severe and thus ultimate visual capabilities may be more limited.

OUTCOMES/RETURN TO PLAY

The outcome of varying sports-related eye injuries obviously depends on the severity of the injury itself. Athletes with small, noncentral corneal abrasions can possibly return to play immediately after evaluation. Similarly, athletes can play with a periorbital contusion provided their eyelids are not swollen shut and they have no concomitant injuries.

Unfortunately, some eye injuries are much more severe and have worse outcomes. A study of ocular trauma in golf showed that of 7 golfers with eye injuries, all 7 required surgical intervention, and 3 required enucleation.[10] In a prospective observational study of 163 soccer-related eye injuries, 22 patients required 42 surgical procedures.[6]

Box 1
Sideline kit

- Pocket-sized Snellen chart (visual acuity is the vital sign for the eye)
- Ophthalmoscope
- Fluorescein stain strips
- Saline drops
- Cobalt blue light
- Topical anesthetic
- Dilating agent

Table 1 Medications	

Anesthetics	• Tetracaine hydrochloride 0.5%, 1%
	  ○ Lasts 15 min, stings
	• Proparacaine hydrochloride 0.5%
	  ○ Lasts 10–15 min, less irritating
	• Note that all anesthetics are toxic to epithelial cells; delay healing

Mydriatics + cycloplegics	• Mydriatics dilate the pupil
	• Cycloplegics additionally paralyze the ciliary muscle (preventing accommodation)
	• Helps visualize fundus, decreases eye pain with iritis, stabilizes blood-ocular barrier in inflammation, prevents formation of posterior synechiae
	• Phenylephrine 2.5%
	  ○ Mydriatic: takes 20 min, lasts 3 h
	• Tropicamide 0.5%, 1%
	  ○ Cycloplegic/mydriatic: takes 20–30 min, lasts 3–6 h

Antibiotics	• Pathogens: Staphylococcus, Streptococcus, Haemophilus
	• Given 4 to 6 times per day, if severe may need fortified or q1 h fluoroquinolone
	  ○ Fortified: tobramycin, gentamicin, vancomycin, cefazolin
	• Ciprofloxacin hydrochloride: Ciloxan
	  ○ Broad-spectrum, especially Staphylococcus, Streptococcus, and Pseudomonas
	  ○ 0.3% solution, 0.3% ointment
	• Erythromycin: AK-mycin, erythromycin, Ilotycin
	  ○ Most gram-positive, diphtheroids, Haemophilus, Actinomyces, Neisseria
	  ○ 0.5% ointment
	• Polymyxin B/trimethoprim: Polytrim
	  ○ Most Staphylococcus, Streptococcus, and Haemophilus
	  ○ 10,000 units, 1 mg/mL solution

Although the retina was successfully reattached in all athletes, only 5 had visual acuities of 20/40 or better and 3 had visual acuity worse than 20/200. Twenty of the patients required hospitalization, with an average stay of 5 days. Of the 45 injured professional players, the average absence time from sport was 15 days; however, this number was increased to 80 days for athletes requiring surgical treatment. One professional player was unable to return to sport, indefinitely.

SIDELINE PREPAREDNESS

With the potential for severe eye injuries during sporting events, team physicians must be prepared. **Box 1** lists items that should be considered when assembling a sideline bag, and **Table 1** outlines some useful medications with which sports medicine physicians should be familiar.

SUMMARY

Blunt visual trauma injuries have the potential to be devastating to the athlete. It is important for sports medicine physicians to be able to clinically recognize the broad range of injuries, treat when able, and refer when appropriate. Although sports in general have an increased risk of ophthalmologic injury, individual sports carry their own risk patterns. Some sports address this with the mandatory use of protective eyewear; however, the current practice or attitude toward protective eyewear is still limited in most sports. The sports medicine physician must be prepared with a basic knowledge of blunt trauma injuries, appropriate tools for evaluation, and understanding of the different ophthalmologic medications available.

REFERENCES

1. Drolsum L. Eye injuries in sports. Scand J Med Sci Sports 1999;9:53–6.
2. Barr A, Baines PS, Desai P, et al. Ocular sports injuries: the current picture. Br J Sports Med 2000;34(6):456–8.
3. Capao Filipe JA, Rocha-Sousa A, Falcao-Reis F, et al. Modern sports eye injuries. Br J Ophthalmol 2003;87(11):1336–9.
4. Sport and Recreational Eye Injuries. Washington, DC: US Consumer Product Safety Commission; 2000.
5. Capao Filipe JA. Soccer (football) ocular injuries: an important eye health problem. Br J Ophthalmol 2004;88(2):159–60.
6. Capao Filipe JA, Fernandes VL, Barros H, et al. Soccer-related ocular injuries. Arch Ophthalmol 2003;121(5):687–94.
7. Bianco M, Vaiano AS, Colella F, et al. Ocular complications of boxing. Br J Sports Med 2005;39(2):70–4 [discussion: 70–4].
8. Giovinazzo VJ, Yannuzzi LA, Sorenson JA, et al. The ocular complications of boxing. Ophthalmology 1987;94(6):587–96.
9. Corrales G, Curreri A. Eye trauma in boxing. Clin Sports Med 2009;28(4): 591–607, vi.
10. Weitgasser U, Wackernagel W, Oetsch K. Visual outcome and ocular survival after sports related ocular trauma in playing golf. J Trauma 2004;56(3):648–50.
11. Hink EM, Oliver SC, Drack AV, et al. Pediatric golf-related ophthalmic injuries. Arch Ophthalmol 2008;126(9):1252–6.
12. American Academy of Family Physicians, American Academy of Pediatrics, American College of Sports Medicine, et al. Eye disorders and vision. In: Roberts W, Bernhardt D, editors. PPE Preparticipation Physical Evaluation. 4th edition. Elk Grove (IL): American Academy of Pediatrics; 2010. p. 80–3.
13. American Academy of Pediatrics Committee on Sports Medicine and Fitness. Protective eyewear for young athletes. Pediatrics 2004;113(3 Pt 1):619–22.
14. Eime RM, Finch CF. Have the attitudes of Australian squash players towards protective eyewear changed over the past decade? Br J Sports Med 2002; 36(6):442–5.
15. Eime R, Finch C, Owen N, et al. Knowledge, beliefs and attitudes of squash venue operators relating to use of protective eyewear. Inj Control Saf Promot 2004;11(1):47–53.
16. Eime R, Finch C, Wolfe R, et al. The effectiveness of a squash eyewear promotion strategy. Br J Sports Med 2005;39(9):681–5.
17. Baker KR, Zimmerman A, Grzybowski DM, et al. Optical quality and impact resistance comparisons of 2 football helmet faceshields. Optometry 2008;79(8):455–63.
18. Vinger PF, Capao Filipe JA. The mechanism and prevention of soccer eye injuries. Br J Ophthalmol 2004;88(2):167–8.
19. Otago L, Adamcewicz E, Eime R, et al. The epidemiology of head, face and eye injuries to female lacrosse players in Australia. Int J Inj Contr Saf Promot 2007; 14(4):259–61.

20. Lincoln AE, Caswell SV, Almquist JL, et al. Effectiveness of the Women's Lacrosse Protective Eyewear Mandate in the Reduction of Eye Injuries. Am J Sports Med 2012;40(3):611–4.
21. Khan MI, Flynn T, O'Connell E, et al. The impact of new regulations on the incidence and severity of ocular injury sustained in hurling. Eye (Lond) 2008;22(4): 475–8.
22. Stevens ST, Lassonde M, deBeaumont L, et al. The effect of visors on head and facial injury in National Hockey League players. J Sci Med Sport 2006;9:238–42.
23. Jones NP. Orbital blowout fractures in sport. Br J Sports Med 1994;28(4):272–5.

Ear Trauma

Kylee Eagles, DO, Laura Fralich, MD*, J. Herbert Stevenson, MD

KEYWORDS

- Ear trauma • External ear • Tympanic membrane • Temporal bone fractures

KEY POINTS

- Understanding basic ear anatomy and function allows an examiner to quickly and accurately identify at-risk structures in patients with head and ear trauma.
- External ear trauma (ie, hematoma and laceration) should be promptly treated with appropriate injury-specific techniques.
- Tympanic membrane (TM) injuries have multiple mechanisms and can often be treated conservatively.
- Temporal bone fractures are a common cause of ear trauma and can be life threatening.
- Facial nerve injuries and hearing loss can occur in ear trauma.

INTRODUCTION

Athletes and active individuals are at risk for ear trauma by virtue of the activities in which they engage. Lacerations of the external ear and TM rupture can occur in everyday life as well. Barotrauma and skull fractures can cause serious damage to the middle and internal ear, leading to problems with balance, tinnitus, facial nerve paralysis, deafness, or even cerebrospinal fluid (CSF) leak and complications, including meningitis. A thorough history and physical examination are essential to diagnosing specific ear trauma injuries along with imaging studies, such as CT or MRI, to confirm diagnostic suspicions. The involvement of ear, nose, and throat (ENT) specialists, otolaryngologist–head and neck surgeons, or neurosurgeons can be crucial to ear trauma outcomes. This article reviews the basic anatomic structures of the external, middle, and internal ear and discusses the causes of specific types of ear trauma that athletes and active individuals are most commonly at risk of experiencing.

EAR ANATOMY REVIEW
External Ear

The external ear (also known as the pinna or auricle) collects sound. The various parts of the external ear includes the helix, antihelix, tragus, antitragus, lobule, and concha. Blood

---

University of Massachusetts Sports Medicine, Department of Family Medicine and Community Health, 275 Nichols Road, 4th Floor, Fitchburg, MA 01420, USA
* Corresponding author.
E-mail address: Laura.Fralich@umassmemorial.org

Clin Sports Med 32 (2013) 303–316
http://dx.doi.org/10.1016/j.csm.2012.12.011
0278-5919/13/$ – see front matter © 2013 Elsevier Inc. All rights reserved.

is supplied to the external ear via the posterior auricular and superficial temporal arteries. The external ear is innervated by the facial nerve, vagus nerve, and great auricular nerve.

The external acoustic meatus is a conduit for sound to the TM (ear drum), a thin, oval membrane that separates the external ear from the middle ear. The TM is responsible for transmission of air vibrations to the auditory ossicles of middle ear. The superior portion of the tympanic membranes is more vascular than its inferior portion. Innervation of the TM includes cranial nerves (CNs) IX (glossopharyngeal), X (vagus), and V3 (auriculotemporal).

Middle Ear

The middle ear is located within the petrous portion of the temporal bone. The tympanic cavity is located within the temporal bone and is directly behind the tympanic membrane, containing the auditory ossicles (small bones of the middle ear): malleus, incus, and stapes. The malleus is attached to the tympanic membrane; its handle presses against the tympanic membrane. The tip of the malleus is known as the umbo and can be seen pushing on the back of TM during otoscopic examination. The chorda tympani nerve crosses over the neck of the malleus and the tensor tympani muscle (innervated by CN V3) inserts into the handle of malleus. The incus is located between the malleus and stapes. The base of the stapes is found within the oval window. The stapedius muscle (innervated by facial nerve) inserts into the neck of stapes and is adjacent to the honeycomb-appearing mastoid cells of the temporal bone. Connecting the middle ear to the nasopharynx is the auditory tube. Also known as the pharyngotympanic tube, this tubular structure of the middle ear equalizes pressures between external ear environment and air of middle ear. Muscles maintaining patency of the auditory tube are part of the soft palate: the tensor veli palatine and levator veli palatine. The blood supply of the auditory tube comes from branches of the external carotid and maxillary artery (including middle meningeal artery).

Internal Ear

The internal ear is responsible for hearing and balance. It is separated from the middle ear by the oval window, which is in direct contact with the stapes. The round window is situated inferior and posterior to the oval window and acts as a secondary TM and allows movement of cochlear fluid necessary for hearing. Within the internal ear, there is a bony labyrinth containing perilymph and a membranous labyrinth suspended within the bony labyrinth containing endolymph. The otic capsule is a bony structure that encloses the structures of the internal ear. The internal acoustic meatus is a narrow opening located within petrous aspect of temporal bone. It is the passageway for the facial (CN VII) and vestibulocochlear nerves (CN VIII). The cochlea is known as the organ of hearing. Shell-shaped with 2.5 turns, the cochlea contains the cochlear duct, which is responsible for hearing (via cochlear and auditory nerves). The internal ear also contains the vestibule, utricle, and saccule, which are essential components of the balance mechanism. The semicircular canals (anterior, posterior, and lateral) are responsible for motion sensation of endolymph, which occurs with head rotation. Each semicircular canal has a duct that is round with an ampulla (swelling at end) and is essential for maintaining balance.

EXTERNAL EAR TRAUMA
Auricular Hematoma

Causes
Sports, such as rugby, water polo, boxing, and wrestling, are associated with increased risk of auricular hematoma compared with other sports. Due to its anatomic

location, the ear is an exposed structure that is at high risk for injury during head trauma. When an ear is struck, shearing forces disrupt the adherence of the perichondrium to the cartilage. In addition to blunt trauma, repeated trauma, such as occurs in wrestling, creates enough force from the friction to separate the perichondrium and the cartilage. This disruption causes the subperichondrial space to fill with blood, which is known as an auricular hematoma. Because cartilage does not have an intrinsic blood supply, it relies on the perichondrium's circulation for a nutritional blood source. When this connection is severed by injury or compressed by a hematoma, the cartilage is at high risk for necrosis and infection. Risk of necrosis is increased when there is an anterior and posterior hematoma surrounding the cartilage of the ear; the hematomas act like a tourniquet and significantly increase the risk of cartilage necrosis. An overlying laceration increases the risk of infection; thus, care must be taken to properly decontaminate the wound and treat with antibiotics if the mechanism of injury increases risk of infection, such as a dog bite or laceration by a dirty object.

Signs and symptoms
A patient reports a traumatic injury or blow to the ear followed by significant swelling or a collection of blood on the outer ear. There is usually pain and pressure. A laceration or inner ear trauma may also be present. It is important to perform a complete examination to rule out any life-threatening injuries and assess for a skull fracture.

Treatment
Treatment of an auricular hematoma involves prompt drainage of the hematoma under sterile technique to minimize risk of infection. There is a choice of either aspirating the hematoma or incision and drainage.[1] For both options, several methods have been proposed (discussed later).

According to Sbaihat and Khatatbeh,[2] using an incision and drainage approach with application of dental rolls has the lowest incidence of recurrence when compared with aspiration or incision and drainage alone. They reported incidences of recurrence of 9.1%, 22.2%, and 37.5% for Incision and drainage with application of dental rolls versus incision and drainage versus aspiration.

Aspiration technique
1. Anesthetize with 1% lidocaine.
2. Sterilize the area with betadine.
3. Insert an 18-gauge needle attached to a 10-mL syringe into the largest area of the hematoma.
4. Aspirate while milking the hematoma with the finger and index finger.
5. Apply pressure for 3 to 5 minutes to the hematoma.
6. If a blood clot remains, then insert a hemostat in the hematoma after making a small incision and break up the clot.
7. Apply a pressure dressing once the entire clot has been removed.
8. Recheck the ear in 24 hours to evaluate for fluid reaccumulation.

Incision and drainage technique
1. Anesthetize with 1% lidocaine.
2. Sterilize the area with betadine.
3. Using a no. 15 blade scalpel, incise the hematoma parallel to the natural skin folds.
4. Completely evacuate the hematoma and irrigate with normal saline.
5. Apply an antibiotic ointment to the incision.
6. Using a 4-0 nylon suture, bring the opposing skin from the incision together, suturing through the cartilage passing the suture around a dental roll that is placed

on the opposite side of the incision. The use of buttons may be used to prevent reformation of the hematoma.
7. Then bring the stitch back through the skin, cartilage, and skin again and through a dental roll on the side of the incision. This creates compression of the drained hematoma area.
8. Prescribe an antistaphylococcal antibiotic.
9. Remove the dental rolls in 1 week.[3]

Complications

The goal of treatment is to prevent abscess formation or permanent deformity of the ear, also known as cauliflower ear, named after the appearance of the ear. Cauliflower ear results from fibrous deposition due to an unevacuated clot.

Prevention

Protective gear should be worn by athletes at risk of receiving a direct blow to the ear. Quick and complete drainage of an auricular hematoma can prevent abscess and scar formation. Follow-up with the patient 24 hours after drainage to assess for reaccumulation of the hematoma.[3]

Return to play

Athletes can return to play (RTP) immediately after evacuation of the hematoma if protective gear is worn and care is taken to minimize risk of infection.

Ear Lacerations

Ear lacerations can be difficult to repair due to the geography of the auricle and the thin skin overlying the cartilage. On a positive note, however, the auricle has a great blood supply and often heals well with minimal risk of infection.

What and when to suture

Small lacerations can be sutured after minimal débridement in an effort to preserve tissue. Reattachment can be achieved as long as a pedicle of skin remains attached to the head. Before repair, irrigate the wound with normal saline.

Helical rim lacerations If the laceration is less than 2 cm, primary closure can be performed. Larger lacerations may require creating a wedge resection or relaxing incisions to allow closure. If the defect is greater than 3 cm, additional tissue (ie, a graft) is required to close the laceration. Try to minimize the number of sutures that go through the cartilage to preserve the blood supply. If there is a V-shaped laceration with a flap, do not approximate the point of the V on the skin flap using a dermal stitch because this places too great a stress on the tissue, creating risk of the suture tearing through or formation of necrosis due to poor blood supply. Instead, use a subcutaneous stitch to approximate the edges.

Total and subtotal avulsion injuries The ability to repair a total or subtotal avulsion injury depends on the extent of tissue loss and bruising, time passed from initial injury, and other injuries that are present. A detached auricle with clean borders should be cleansed in cold clean saline as soon as possible and then placed in heparinized Ringer lactate solution. The ear must be reattached within 3 hours of the initial avulsion. Athletes must not have other injuries that preclude the use of heparin. Clean and débride the avulsed edges while taking care to avoid excising more than 1 mm of tissue. Anesthetize with 1% or 2% lidocaine without epinephrine. Reapproximate with interrupted sutures.[4]

Suture material

6-0 Nonabsorbable monofilament suture.[3]

A helpful way to create a sterilized field during an ear laceration repair is discussed later.

Indications for referral

Refer for avulsion injuries or lacerations requiring a higher level of expertise to repair.

Complications

With large laceration and avulsion injuries, there can be blood loss significant enough to necessitate a blood transfusion. Failure to cover cartilage with skin can result in chondritis and subsequent ear deformities.[3]

Return to play

Small lacerations may return once repair is made and hemostasis is obtained with appropriate protection. Larger repairs and avulsion injuries require full tissue healing before RTP, particularly if there is a risk of reinjury. Advise athletes on proper protection of the ear and prevention of infection.

Tympanic Membrane Perforation

Causes

The TM is a 3-layered membrane that lies in the middle ear. TM perforation (TMP) results from several different mechanisms of trauma. Perforation or rupture can occur from acoustic trauma, barotrauma, foreign object trauma, or a powerful slap or explosion.[5] Middle ear pressure can also increase from otitis media and result in perforation. Middle ear pressure is equilibrated by the tensor veli palatini muscle and the salpingopharyngeus muscle. Sports with higher risk for TMP include scuba diving, surfing, wrestling, boxing, mixed martial arts, and diving. Temporal bone basilar skull fracture has a 50% association with TMP. Approximately one-third of severe head trauma cases have an associated TMP. Crossing the middle ear are the ossicular chain and the facial nerve; thus, when there is TMP, injury to these structures must be assessed as well.[6]

Signs and symptoms

Sudden hearing loss is the primary initial complaint after TMP has occurred. Other signs are dizziness, ear pain, tinnitus, nausea, and, in severe cases, weakness in the face. Additional symptoms are bleeding, otorrhea, rhinorrhea, imbalance, or infection. When assessing patients, first ensure they are stable and have no life-threatening injuries. Then proceed to the otoscopic examination to assess the extent of damage. Document what percent of the TM has been perforated, look for other signs of trauma to the ear, and assess for infection or bleeding in the ear. It is also imperative to assess for any signs of skull fracture, such as the presence of a Battle sign, which can occur anywhere for 6 hours to 2 days after injury. Evaluate hearing using the Rinne and Weber tests. If available, use an audiometer for more accurate assessment of hearing loss. TMP results in a conductive hearing loss.

Treatment

Recovery from TMP relies primarily on allowing the TM to attempt to heal itself. The initial role is to determine when to offer supportive care in the way of pain management and infection prevention versus the need to refer to otolaryngology.

Indications for referral to otolaryngology[6]
- Hearing loss greater than 40 dB on audiometry testing or subjective decreased perception of speech, marked asymmetry in hearing, or persisting feelings of ear fullness
- Basilar skull fracture
- Otorrhea or rhinorrhea
- Facial nerve paralysis/paresis
- Vestibular symptoms, such as nausea, vomiting, nystagmus, ataxia

Indications for hospital admission
- Basillar skull fracture
- Ossicular disruption
- Acute traumatic facial nerve paralysis
- Perilymph fistula
- Refractory nausea/vomiting necessitating intravenous rehydration or antiemetics

Pain management

A dry warm compress over the ear can alleviate pain in addition to over-the-counter analgesics, such as acetaminophen. If there is concern about head trauma in association with the TMP, avoid the use of nonsteroidal anti-inflammtory drugs because they can increase the risk of intracranial bleeding.

Infection prevention

It is important to prevent water from entering the inner ear because this increases the risk of infection. Therefore, ear protection is needed when showering. Swimming is prohibited until the TM has healed. If the wound is contaminated, treat with ofloxacin otic drops. Place 5 drops in the ear, twice a day for 3 to 5 days.[6]

Re-evaluate 4 weeks after the injury to re-assess hearing with audiometry. If there is persistent perforation or hearing loss, refer to otolaryngology.

Complications

Otitis media, mastoiditis, and permanent hearing loss are potential complications of TMP.

Prevention

TMP can be prevented by wearing protective headgear during sports in which an athlete is at high risk for head trauma, such as wrestling, boxing, and mixed martial arts. For underwater sports, it is recommended to ascend to the surface slowly to allow the inner ear to equilibrate. Avoid placing any foreign objects in the ear. Wear earplugs or a noise-canceling headset if participating in a sporting event, such as hunting.

Return to play

A TMP usually heals in 4 to 8 weeks. RTP after a TMP injury depends on the sport. Swimmers, divers, and surfers should not RTP until the TM has fully healed. If there is an associated skull fracture or other trauma, the athlete cannot RTP until recovered from those injuries. The athlete must have return of balance before RTP. Other considerations, such as degree of hearing loss, depend on the sport being resumed.

MIDDLE EAR TRAUMA
Otic Barotrauma

Causes
Otic barotrauma (aerotitis media or barotitis media) is defined as ear pain and/or traumatic injury to the TM caused by rapid changes in pressure. Most often caused by flying (particularly during descent); other activities increasing the risk of otic barotrauma include scuba diving and water-skiing (hitting external ear on the water during fall). Pressure differences between air in the middle ear and that of the external environment can cause traumatic inflammation and/or rupture of the tympanic membrane.[7] If the Eustachian tube is not patent (ie, ear or sinus infection), pressure builds and stresses the TM (retracts or bulges).

Signs and symptoms
Patients may complain of otalgia, a sensation of ear fullness, vertigo, or hearing loss (conductive or sensorineural). Rupture of the TM, ecchymosis, and hematoma of the TM (Image 1) or a perilymphatic fistula may also develop or be evident.

Diagnosis
A history of recent air travel or diving often raises suspicion for otic barotrauma. An otoscopic examination of the ear reveals TM hematoma or fluid as well as possible TM rupture. The hearing examination can indicate conductive hearing loss or sensorineural hearing loss if inner ear is involved.

Complications
The prognosis is often good and patients can be monitored. Hearing loss (conductive or sensorineural) and perilymphatic fistula can occur, however, prompting evaluation by an ENT specialist.

Treatment
Equalizing ear pressure by popping the ears is often used. This can be accomplished by chewing gum, yawning, swallowing, or using the Valsalva maneuver. Using a nasal decongestant (oral or spray) before travel or diving to improve Eustachian tube function may be useful and is somewhat controversial. If TM perforation has occurred, monitor for 3 months and then refer for surgical repair if not healed. If there is an identifiable TM hematoma or fluid, patients can be monitor or referred for myringotomy to drain fluid.[8]

Prevention
Avoid air travel or diving if nasal congestion, ear infection, severe allergy symptoms, or Eustachian tube dysfunction is present. Also avoid rapid changes in atmospheric pressure (ascend and descend slowly) when flying or scuba diving.

Return to play
Individuals should not return to water sports until the TM has completely healed. It is safe to fly in an airplane with a ruptured tympanic membrane.[7,9] Patients who have undergone surgical repair of the TM (ie, myringoplasty), however, should consult with a surgeon before flying or returning to water sports.

Basilar Skull and Temporal Bone Fractures

Causes
Basilar skull and temporal bone fractures are caused by falls or severe head trauma (ie, motor vehicle accident, assault, or blunt trauma). Individuals involved in sports, such as motorcross and racecar driving, are at increased risk for these types of

fractures, as are people who skateboard and ride bicycles or motorcycles. These fractures go through the base of the skull or temporal bones that house the middle ear, internal ear, and facial nerve and can extend to the inner ear and petrous portion of the temporal bone (Image 2). Temporal bone fractures are often identified as longitudinal (most common), transverse, or oblique fractures.

Signs and symptoms
Patients who sustain a basilar skull fracture or temporal bone fracture can experience loss of consciousness, dizziness, vertigo, hearing loss (due to blood accumulation in the middle ear or disruption of the ossicles and cochlea), facial paresis or paralysis[10] (geniculate ganglion involvement), hemotympanum, or TM rupture. Clinicians may find postauricular ecchymoses, known as Battle sign or raccoon eyes, terms for ecchymoses under the eyes. Patients may also experience blood or CSF from the nose and/or ears (often from temporal bone fractures).

Diagnosis
A history of head trauma (often blunt or high-energy mechanism) should significantly raise suspicion of a basilar skull or temporal bone fracture. Examination findings are discussed previously. High-resolution head CT is the gold standard for diagnosis although MRI can be useful for identifying CN injuries and magnetic resonance angiography for vascular damage (ie, internal carotid artery). It is also important to assess hearing and facial nerve function.

Prognosis
Prognosis of basilar skull and temporal bone fractures varies based on the degree of injury. If a transverse temporal bone fracture is identified, severe brain injury has also likely occurred and the prognosis is guarded.

Complications
Complications of basilar skull and temporal bone fractures include facial paralysis, hearing loss, CSF leak and/or fistula, encephalocele, cholesteatoma, meningitis, severe brain injury sequelae, carotid artery injury, and death.

Treatment
Observation of persons with basilar skull fractures can be a reasonable option, particularly if neurologically stable. Surgical intervention is used in more complicated or emergent cases of basilar or temporal bone fractures, such as brain herniation, intracranial bleeding, immediate or persistent facial nerve paralysis, hearing loss, or persistent CSF leak (longer than 2 weeks). The use of prophylactic antibiotics is controversial and generally not used. Steroids have been used to treat acute hearing loss and facial nerve injuries.[11]

Return to play
Individuals who have sustained basilar or temporal bone fractures should discuss returning to activities with their doctor and should not RTP until fractures have completely healed.

INTERNAL EAR TRAUMA
Inner Ear Decompression Sickness

Causes
Also known as the staggers, inner ear (vestibulocochlear apparatus) decompression sickness is a condition affecting scuba divers in which gas bubble formation occurs in the inner ear when ascending from a deep-water dive (usually greater

than 100 feet). Scuba divers who do not practice proper decompression techniques while ascending in the water or who use a helium-oxygen mixture in their scuba tank (instead of nitrogen-oxygen) can experience inner ear decompression sickness; helium is known to diffuse from the middle ear to the inner ear across the round window membrane, possibly predisposing divers to inner ear bubble formation.

Signs/symptoms
Divers who suffer from inner ear decompression sickness may complain of vertigo, tinnitus, nausea, vomiting, or hearing loss in one or both ears. Individuals may also have difficulty maintaining proper balance while ambulating due to vestibulocochlear apparatus dysfunction, hence the staggers.

Diagnosis
Diagnosis can be made by reports of recent deep water diving, identifying signs and symptoms of inner ear decompression sickness, and observing signs of possible barotrauma on otoscopic examination. Further work-up may also reveal a patent ductus arteriosus, patent foramen ovale, or right-to-left heart shunt.[9]

Complications
Permanent vestibulocochlear damage, hearing loss, and TM barotrauma.

Treatment
Hyperbaric oxygen therapy and/or monitoring for resolution of symptoms.

Prevention
Limiting dive depths to less than 100 feet is a significant way to reduce the risk of inner ear decompression sickness. The use of a nitrogen-oxygen mixture in scuba tanks also helps prevent occurrence. Finally, encouraging divers to practice proper decompression techniques during ascent in the water is important.[8]

Return to play
An individual's diving fitness should be assessed by a physician who specializes in dive medicine before being cleared to dive. Persons may return to diving if they are deemed fit by a dive medicine specialist, if neurologic and cardiologic examinations are normal, if asymptomatic, and if the TM has completely healed (if initially damaged).

Blast Ear Injury

Causes
The ear is susceptible to blast injuries involving the tympanic membrane; middle ear structures, such as the auditory ossicles and/or the internal ear; and the external ear (ie, flying debris). Blast ear injuries can occur on the job, battlefield, indoors, or outdoors and are more severe when there is less reflection or obstruction of the blast energy wave en route to the TM.

Signs and symptoms
Tinnitus, otalgia, bilateral or unilateral hearing loss (sensorineural, conductive, or mixed), and vertigo are common complaints. Unilateral or bilateral TM perforation may also occur.

Diagnosis
Otoscopic examination may be normal or show evidence of external ear or TM damage. It is important to assess both conductive and sensorineural hearing. Head CT or MRI may be used to determine the severity of blast trauma.

Complications

Cholesteatoma formation, which can erode surrounding bone, meningitis, abscess formation, progressively worsening ability to hear or persistent hearing loss, CN dysfunction, and balance problems.[12]

Treatment

Consultation with audiologists, ENTs, and/or otolaryngologists regarding blast ear injuries, particularly if there is damage to the TM and/or hearing loss. Surgical intervention may be warranted.

Prevention

Wearing ear protection can prevent blast injuries to the ears.

Return to play

Blast ear injuries may result in complications requiring individuals to retire early, be discharged from the military, or become legally disabled. Return to activity or RTP depends on the extent of individual ear injury and if patients can safely perform preinjury tasks. Ear protection may also be warranted.

Otic Capsule Injury

Causes

Otic capsule injuries are rare, caused by disruption or fracture of the otic capsule, the bony structure that surrounds the inner ear. This can occur due to a fracture of the temporal bone or occiput by blunt trauma and/or a fracture that travels directly into the otic capsule and damages the cochlea and semicircular canals.[11]

Signs/symptoms

Otic capsule injuries can be accompanied by a skull fracture (with or without Battle and raccoon signs), TM perforation, hemotympanum, otorrhea, facial paralysis, vertigo, nystagmus, or hearing loss.

Diagnosis

A history of head trauma is common. Use of head CT or head MRI (noncontrast/contrast-enhanced MR cisternography to look at inner ear structures if fistula suspected) is also used. Audiogram assessment is another useful confirmatory diagnostic tool.

Complications

There are many potential complications of otic capsule injuries due to the fragility of the structures the capsule surrounds and its proximity to other cranial structures. These complications include facial paralysis, CSF leak, meningitis, meningocele, hearing loss, epidural hematoma, subacrachnoid hemorrhage, and encephalocele.[11]

Treatment

Surgical repair of the capsule by a head and neck surgeon or close, conservative monitoring by ENT are treatment options based on severity of injury, concomitant injuries, or associated complications.

Return to play

Dependent on extent of damage and risk of future injury.

Cochlear Concussion

Causes

Also known as an inner ear concussion or labyrinth concussion, a cochlear concussion involves tearing of the membranous labyrinth causing damage to the cochlea (shell-shaped structure of bony labyrinth that contains the membranous labyrinth's cochlear duct, responsible for hearing). Damage to the cochlea is caused by a traumatic blow to the head but not severe enough to cause a fracture.[12]

Signs ad symptoms
Mild to complete hearing loss, vertigo, tinnitus, and facial nerve paralysis are potential signs and symptoms of cochlear concussion. Patients can have a normal-appearing TM although hemotympanum and TM perforation can occur.

Diagnosis
A history of head trauma is important for diagnosing cochlear concussion. Otoscopic evaluation and CN examinations may be normal. Head CT or MRI can definitively identify the injury.

Treatment
It is important for patients with cochlear concussions to be evaluated by an ENT specialist and/or neurosurgery, promptly if hearing loss or facial nerve paralysis exist.

Complications
Complications of cochlear concussion include hearing loss, facial nerve paralysis, and disequilibrium.

Return to play
Dependent on extent of damage and risk of future injury.

Oval Window Trauma/Perilymphatic Fistula

Causes
Trauma to the oval window, which is covered by a membrane and transmits vibrations from the stapes in the air-filled middle ear into the fluid-filled inner ear, is often caused by barotrauma (ie, flying and scuba diving).[9] A perilymphatic fistula (also known as labyrinth fistula) is an abnormal communication between the perilymphatic space of the inner ear and the middle ear or mastoid (can be difficult to diagnose).

Signs and symptoms
Nausea, vomiting, vertigo, imbalance, sensorineural deafness, tinnitus, and a sensation of ear fullness.

Diagnosis
Otoscopic examination may be normal. To confirm oval window trauma or the presence of a perlymphatic fistula, head CT or MRI is obtained. A noncontrast/contrast-enhanced cisternography can assist in early diagnosis and management of suspected fistulas. Exploratory tympanotomy is an alternative method to diagnose such trauma or fistula formation.[9]

Complications
A labyrinth fistula and perilymphatic leakage can permanently damage the inner ear.

Treatment
Tympanotomy can be performed to assist with healing. A fistula can be surgically closed with fat grafting as well.

Return to play
Dependent on extent of damage and risk of future injury.

Facial Nerve Injury

The facial nerve, also known as CN VII, innervates the muscles of facial expression and the middle ear. It is also responsible for taste on the anterior two-thirds of the tongue and sensation of the external ear as well as lacrimation and salivation. The facial nerve and its branches are susceptible to injury from head and/or ear trauma because of its course through the skull, including the internal acoustic meatus, temporal bone, stylomastoid foramen, and parotid gland. It is the most commonly injured CN.

Causes

Temporal bone fractures are the most common cause of traumatic injury to the facial nerve; transverse temporal bone fractures account for more facial nerve injuries than longitudinal fractures.[10,11] Motor vehicle accidents, extreme sports, falls, and gunshot wounds can result in traumatic ear and subsequent facial nerve injuries. Edema surrounding/compressing the nerve can mimic a facial nerve injury.

Signs and symptoms

Unilateral or bilateral facial paresis (weakness) or paralysis with facial asymmetry is seen with facial nerve injuries. These symptoms may have a delayed onset, particularly after temporal bone trauma.[11] Ability to taste, lacrimation, and salivation may also be impaired depending on the location of the nerve injury.

Diagnosis

High-resolution head CT scanning with axial and coronal images is the diagnostic tool of choice for evaluating the facial nerve in temporal bone trauma. MRI can also be used to identify CN injuries. Electroneuronography testing can also be performed to assess facial nerve conductivity; this is generally done within 2 to 3 weeks of injury.[11] The House-Brackmann classification system is often used to grade the severity of facial nerve injuries: grade 1 = normal, grade 2 = mild dysfunction, grade 3 = moderate dysfunction, grade 4 = moderately severe dysfunction, grade 5 = severe dysfunction, and grade 6 = total paralysis.

Complications

Late-onset facial nerve paralysis can occur. Permanent partial or complete loss of facial nerve function.

Treatment

Surgery (ie, decompression or other) is often considered for patients with immediate facial paralysis after injury, nerve paralysis that does not resolve, or those with no evidence of nerve stimulus conductivity. Concomitant injuries, such as temporal bone disruption, may also warrant surgical intervention. Steroids have also been used in the acute setting of facial nerve injury.[11]

Return to play

Patients with facial nerve injuries can often return to activity as tolerated once cleared by a physician.

Hearing Loss

Causes

Skull fractures, particularly those of the temporal bone, as well as blast ear injuries, blunt head trauma, and direct ear trauma can result in hearing loss. Sensorineural hearing loss is often the result of injury to the internal ear (ie, cochlea) or the vestibulocochlear nerve (CN VIII), whereas conductive hearing loss typically occurs due to damage of the TM and/or middle ear (ie, ossicles). Mixed hearing loss is a result of injuries to both auditory components. Transverse temporal bone fractures are more commonly responsible for sensorineural hearing loss and longitudinal fractures are more frequently associated with conductive and mixed hearing loss.[11]

Signs and symptoms
Partial or complete hearing loss, evidence of head injury, tinnitus, vertigo, otalgia, hemotympanum, TM perforation, difficulty with speech.

Diagnosis
It is important to assess auditory acuity of the patient with ear trauma. In the acute setting, hearing loss can be mistaken for unconsciousness or give the impression of a concussed and disoriented patient. Simply asking patients if they can hear the questioner is the most basic diagnostic test. A tuning fork (Weber and Rinne tests) can be used to assess for conductive and sensorineural hearing loss and audiometry can be used to identify severity of hearing loss. High-resolution head CT scans of the temporal bones can also be used to visualize structural damage of the ear structures.

Complications
Permanent hearing loss.

Treatment
Hearing loss spontaneously resolves in the majority of cases. Sensorineural hearing loss due to internal ear injury has a worse prognosis, however, than conductive hearing loss and persists despite treatment. Corticosteroids have been used to acutely treat sensorineural damage without good long-term results. Cochlear implants can be beneficial for some patients. Surgery to repair damage to the external and middle ear structures can be delayed until surrounding edema and bleeding have resolved. Hearing aids provide amplification of sound and can improve auditory acuity.[10,11]

Prevention
Use protective equipment, such as helmets, seatbelts, ear protection, and other devices, to minimize head and ear trauma.

Return to play
Athletes and active individuals may RTP depending on the extent of hearing loss, ear damage, and risks associated with specific activities.

REFERENCES

1. Macdonald D, et al. Case presentation: a novel way of treating acute cauliflower ear in a professional rugby player. Br J Sports Med 2005;39(6):e29. http://dx.doi.org/10.1136/bjsm.2004.015115.
2. Ahmad S, Sbaihat, Ahmed S, MD, Khatatbeh, Wesam J, MD. Treatment of Auricular Hematoma Using Dental Rolls Splints. Journal of the Royal Medical Services June 2011;Vol. 18. No. 2.
3. King, Christopher and Henretig, Fred. Textbook of Emergency Pediatric Procedures. Chapter 55. External Ear Procedures. Lippincott and WIlliams; 2008. p. 594–8.
4. Patil R. Easy way of keeping hairs away while suturing ear lacerations. Indian J Plast Surg 2011;44(3):531. http://dx.doi.org/10.4103/0970-0358.90860.
5. Afolabi, Olushola, et al. Traumatic Tympanic Membrane perforation: An aetiological profile. BMC Res Notes 2009;2:232. Published online 2009 November 21. http://dx.doi.org/10.1186/1756-0500-2-232.

6. Malloy, Kelly MD and Hollander, Judd MD. Assessment and management of auricle (ear) lacerations. Up to date. 2012.
7. Mirza S, Richardson H. Otic barotrauma from air travel. J Laryngol Otol 2005; 119(5):366–70.
8. Klingmann C, Paetorius M, Baumann I, Plinkert PK. Barotrauma and decompression illness of the inner ear: 46 cases during treatment and follow up. Otol Neurotol 2007;28(4):447–54.
9. Park GY, Byun H, Moon IJ, Hong SH, Cho YS, Chung WH. Effects of early surgical exploration in suspected barotraumatic perilymph fistulas. Clin Exp Otorhinolaryngol 2012;5(2):74–80.
10. Patel A, Groppo E. Management of temporal bone trauma. Craniomaxillofac Trauma Reconstr 2010;3(2):105–13.
11. Nash JJ, Friedland DR, Boorsma KJ, Rhee JS. Management and outcomes of facial paralysis from intratemporal blunt trauma: a systematic review. Laryngoscope 2010;120(7):1397–404.
12. Darley DS, Kellman RM. Otologic considerations of blast injury. Disaster Med Public Health Prep 2010;4(2):145–52.

Muscle Contusion (Thigh)

Thomas H. Trojian, MD[a,b,c],*

KEYWORDS

- Quadriceps contusion • Immobilization • Myositis ossificans
- Compartment syndrome • Muscle repair

KEY POINTS

- Thigh contusions are a common injury in sports that can cause prolonged disability if not treated correctly.
- The knee needs to be placed in 120° of flexion for 24 hours, with limited use of nonsteroidal anti-inflammatory drugs for the first 48 to 72 hours.
- Complications such as myositis ossificans and compartment syndrome need to be considered.

INTRODUCTION

Muscle injuries are common problem in sports, with contusions being reported as 12.1% of all injuries.[1] Muscle contusions are more frequently seen in males (15.1%) than in females (6.3%).[1] Sports such as American football, soccer, and softball have a higher frequency of muscle injuries.[2] In high school sports, boys are more likely to suffer contusions than girls.[2] Contusion injuries are more likely (per athletic exposure) to occur during games than during practice.[3] The locations of contusions are not listed by body parts in epidemiology studies, but contusions are reported to comprise 14.2% of all thigh injuries in high school sports (15.8% in boys and 11.2% in girls)[1] and 19% of all muscle injuries in professional soccer.[3] Jackson and Feagin[4] reported that the average return to duty without proper treatment of thigh contusions was 45 days. Therefore thigh contusions are a common problem in sports, which can cause prolonged disability without proper treatment.

PATHOPHYSIOLOGY

A thigh contusion occurs when a compressive force applied to the quadriceps muscle is not dispersed, and the muscle and underlying tissue is squeezed into the femur. The myofibers and capillaries rupture. Because the thigh has a large potential space,

a Orthopaedics, UCHC/NEMSI, Farmington, CT, USA; b Family Medicine, UCHC, Farmington, CT, USA; c Department of Athletics, University of Connecticut, Storrs, CT, USA
* 99 Woodland Street, Hartford, CT 06105.
E-mail address: ttrojian@uchc.edu

Clin Sports Med 32 (2013) 317–324
http://dx.doi.org/10.1016/j.csm.2012.12.009
0278-5919/13/$ – see front matter © 2013 Elsevier Inc. All rights reserved.

a large hematoma can develop; therefore, proper treatment from the beginning is important.[5]

When a thigh contusion occurs the muscle heals by a repair process, not a regenerative process as occurs in bone.[5,6] The tissue does not return to the original state, and scar is present. Repair occurs in 3 overlapping phases: (1) destruction phase (0–7 days), (2) repair phase (7–21 days), and (3) remodeling phase (>21 days).[6]

1. Destruction phase. This phase is characterized by the rupture and ensuing necrosis of the myofibers and formation of a hematoma. Macrophages clean up damaged cells. Fibroblasts lay down type-3 collagen to form scar. Myosatellite cells, small mononuclear progenitor cells with virtually no cytoplasm found in mature muscle, which are precursors to skeletal muscle cells, give rise to satellite cells or differentiated skeletal muscle cells in the regenerative zone. By day 5 the scar is denser and myotubes are formed.
2. Repair phase. This phase consists in the phagocytosis of the necrotized tissue, regeneration of the myofibers, and concomitant formation of connective scar tissue. There is vascular ingrowth. By day the scar starts to break down. By day 14 the scar is reduced. By day 21 myofibers are interlaced, with little scar intermixed.
3. Remodeling phase. During this period maturation of the regenerated myofibers, retraction and reorganization of the scar tissue, and recovery of the functional capacity of the muscle occurs.[6]

The repair of the skeletal muscle, including the formation of a fibrotic scar following injury, depends on numerous factors.[7] The activity of 2 cell types, myosatellite cells and fibroblasts, may be the determining variable in deciding the ultimate fate of the injured skeletal muscle. Myosatellite cells become myoblasts and repair muscle by fusing with injured, but surviving myofibers, or by de novo formation of new myotubes to form new myofibers.[7] After injury, fibroblasts proliferate in the area of the damaged muscle and begin to produce a collagen-rich extracellular matrix to restore the muscle's connective tissue framework.[8,9] Activated fibroblasts also release chemoattractants, which recruit additional fibroblasts and inflammatory cells to the injured tissue.[10,11] Excess proliferation and activation of fibroblasts can lead to unwanted unnecessary fibrosis and dense scar tissue, which can obstruct the muscle's regenerative process and result in incomplete recovery.[12]

One of the important chemoattractants is transforming growth factor (TGF)-β1, which comes from macrophages and is responsible for the increased production of collagen and extracellular matrix. Interferon-γ has been shown to not only downregulate endogenous collagen expression but also to effectively block TGF-β1–mediated increases in collagen protein levels. Increased interferon-γ induces SMAD-7, which, via a negative feedback loop, reduces TGF-β1.[11]

PHYSICAL EXAMINATION

The mechanism of injury is a compressive force to the thigh. This force usually causes disability that prevents further play, but frequently the injury can be less severe and will not limit the athlete until after completion of play, when the bleeding and swelling has reached a tipping point. History of trauma with pain and limp are very common. If treatment is delayed or the injury is severe, compartment syndrome needs to be considered.

Certain features are very important in the history and physical examination of thigh muscle contusion. Alonso and colleagues have developed a prognostic algorithm to determine the number of days until full training. From the history, the ability to play following injury (yes or no beyond 5 minutes) and the number of hours between injury and presentation for treatment are important. Physical examination should record degrees of knee flexion on both legs, firmness rating from −5 to +5 of injured muscle, and circumference of thigh at suprapatelllar border in both legs.

$$DFT = 0.05 \ (DROM) + 0.73 \ (FR) + 1.34 \ (DC1) - 3.21 \ (Able \ to \ play) - 0.04 \ (hours) + 4.32^{13}$$

where DFT = days between presentation for treatment and return to full training, DROM = uninjured-injured interlimb difference in knee flexion range (degrees), FR = firmness rating of the injured muscle on −5 to +5 scale, DC1 = injured-uninjured circumference difference at the suprapatellar border (cm), Able to play = ability to carry on playing following injury (0 = No, 1 = Yes), and hours = hours between injury and presentation.

Compartment syndrome caused by bleeding into the thigh compartments needs to be considered. The thigh is divided into anterior and posterior compartments by the medial and lateral intermuscular septa. The anterior compartment contains the femoral nerve, which innervates all of the muscles of the compartment, and provides sensation over the area of the knee, medial leg, and foot via the saphenous nerve.[14] Intracompartment pressures are indicated if signs of compartment syndrome are found (pain, pulselessness, paresthesia, paralysis). In thigh contusions that developed anterior thigh compartment syndromes, Mithofer and colleagues[15] reported that an excessively painful, tensely swollen thigh was seen in all patients; with pain with passive stretch in 100%; 60% of patients had paresthesia, 7% had pulselessness, and 40% had paralysis. Compartment pressures of 30 mm Hg or higher are suggested for surgical intervention.[14]

IMAGING

Ultrasonography has several important potential advantages over magnetic resonance imaging (MRI), such as superior spatial resolution, cost, convenience, portability, and dynamic evaluation of the injury.[16] In a study by Megliola and colleagues[17] where ultrasonography was compared with MRI, there were 8 minor and 29 severe contusions (functional loss, strength reduction, muscle hypertonia, and increased muscle volume proportional to pain intensity) examined by ultrasonography performed after the injury (6–72 hours after injury) and by MRI within 5 days. Ultrasonography identified all of the 29 severe contusions and 7 of the 8 minor contusions, with the extra days MRI was capable of detecting swelling and muscle injury that may have been missed on the initial ultrasonogram.[17] Therefore, ultrasonography appears to be an equivalent method of identifying muscle contusion injury, and has the advantage of allowing aspiration of hematoma and serial evaluation.[18,19] Ultrasonography should thus be considered the first-line imaging tool for thigh contusion.[17]

On ultrasonography, thigh contusion is characterized by discontinuity of normal muscle architecture with ill-defined hyperechogenicity. This appearance may cross fascial boundaries, different to that of muscle strains. MRI typically demonstrates a feathery appearance of diffuse edema on short-tau inversion recovery and fat-suppressed T2-weighted images. Hematoma will be hypoechogenic on ultrasonography but will show an increased signal on MRI. Acute hematomas (<48 hours) are typically isointense on T1-weighted images, and subacute hematomas (<30 days) appear hyperintense relative to muscle on both T1-weighted and fluid-sensitive sequences, secondary to methemoglobin accumulation.[18,20]

TREATMENT

It is important to approach treatment of thigh contusions in a staged manner. Treatment should be based on the time from injury.

1. Immediate care: control of the bleeding and minimizing the size of the secondary area of injury
2. Acute phase: restoration of pain-free range of motion
3. Subacute phase: functional rehabilitation
4. Long term: gradual return to normal activity

Immediate Care

As soon as the athlete can no longer participate in sport, the knee of the contused thigh should be immediately flexed painlessly and immobilized in 120° of flexion with an elastic wrap. It is important to limit the hematoma by controlling bleeding through maintaining knee flexion. The knee can be maintained in 120° of knee flexion with an elastic wrap or an adjustable range-of-motion brace set at 120° of flexion.[21] The patient will need to use crutches, and should maintain this position of knee flexion for 24 hours.[4,21–23] Nonsteroidal anti-inflammatory drugs (NSAIDs) should be administered for the first 48 to 72 hours only.[24]

Acute Phase

After the brace is discontinued, active pain-free range-of-motion stretching should take place several times a day. Cryotherapy should be used with continuation of NSAIDs until 48 to 72 hours.[24] Crutches are continued until there is pain-free knee flexion equal to the uninjured side, and size and firmness of the contracted quadriceps equal to the uninjured side.

Subacute Phase

The athlete should be able to perform the activities needed for the sport, and should be required to wear, for the remainder of the season, a basic thigh pad modified with a ring-shaped pad to prevent recurrent trauma to the area of the contusion.[21]

Return to sport should not be allowed without[21]:

1. Pain-free knee flexion
2. Quadriceps size and firmness equal to the uninjured side
3. Regaining the mobility and agility unique to the specific sport
4. Wearing, for the remainder of the season, a basic thigh pad modified with a ring-shaped pad to prevent recurrent trauma to the area of the contusion

ADJUNCTIVE TREATMENTS

NSAIDs appear to have a paradoxic effect on the healing of muscle injuries, with early signs of improvement and subsequent late impairment in functional capacity and histology.[25] NSAID use in the first 3 days appears not to have a detrimental effect, but continued use appears to affect healing in a negative manner.[24] Animal studies show no difference between NSAIDs and acetaminophen.[26]

Cryotherapy for sport-related injuries needs further research as a possible treatment to prevent secondary damage.[24] The effects and benefits of cryotherapy have not been fully elucidated.[27] Cryotherapy is able to modulate the oxidative damage, possibly by its capacity to limit the intensity of the inflammatory response and attenuate the impairment of the mitochondrial function, thereby preserving the morphology of skeletal muscle.[28] It been shown that cryotherapy is associated with a significantly smaller hematoma between the ruptured myofiber stumps, less inflammation and tissue necrosis, and a slight accelerated early regeneration response.[29,30]

The effects of corticosteroids might be different between muscle strain and contusion. Corticosteroids have been shown to slow healing in contusion injuries by delaying the clearance of debris at the site of injury and prolonging the muscle regenerative process and recovery of muscle strength.[24,31] Glucocorticosteroids have an effect on macrophages, altering their function,[24] but this process may be different in muscle strains,[32] where early administration of corticosteroids has been shown to be beneficial.

Suramin is a heparin analogue that can bind to heparin-binding proteins and inhibit the effect of growth factors, including TGF-β1, by competitively binding to the growth factor receptors.[33] Suramin is not part of the current standard treatment in humans, and there are many side effects apparent in its use as an antiparasitic and antineoplastic agent.[34] Suramin injected in animals at 2 weeks after contusion injury showed increased strength with more regenerating myofibers and less fibrotic scar at 4 weeks.[35] Further research is needed before it should be used in humans with thigh contusions.

COMPLICATIONS
Myositis Ossificans

The incidence of myositis ossificans (MO) after muscle contusion has been reported to be 9% to 17%.[23] The incidence varies with severity, with 4% occurrence in mild contusions and 18% in severe contusions.[4] Initially MO on examination consists of a doughy mass that gradually becomes indurated[36]; this finding may be found in only a few hours. If the symptoms increase 2 to 3 weeks after the trauma, with the development of more induration and loss of range of motion in the affected thigh, MO should be considered. Radiographs and ultrasonography are warranted, and the earliest radiographic changes, a soft-tissue mass that may be accompanied by faint periosteal bone formation, occurs within 7 to 14 days. The radiologic findings evolve as the lesion matures, with the mineralization greatest at the periphery of the lesion and the central zone being relatively radiolucent. At about 10 weeks onward, radiographs will show a zoning pattern of peripheral maturation, producing an "eggshell" appearance. By 4 to 6 months, the lesion usually gives the appearance of mature lamellar bone and may begin to show absorption.

The different stages of MO are detectable with ultrasonography, and initial findings may precede plain radiographs. The precalcified stage can cause diagnostic problems, because MO is not always connected to a recent trauma and can resemble sarcoma.[37] A solid-appearing mass with detectable Doppler signal throughout, especially at the periphery, is found on ultrasonographic examination. Unlike sarcoma, the size of the lesion increases more rapidly. Sarcoma typically is slow growing unless there is intralesional hemorrhage, which can be identified on ultrasonography. Later, MO may appear as a hypoechoic or heterogeneous mass, with sheets of echogenic calcifications, which are usually peripherally oriented. The mass may also demonstrate marked vascularity of the rim and central zone on Doppler imaging at this stage, differentiating the lesion from an intramuscular abscess. Finally, as the lesion matures, acoustic shadowing caused by peripheral ossification is seen.[37]

On MRI the initial findings are ill defined,[38] because the MO lesion starts as isointense to muscle on T1-weighted images and heterogeneous on T2-weighted images. There is often a large area of surrounding edema, with concern for a neoplasm. The lesion becomes better defined with maturity, with fat signal intensity from ossification on both T1-weighted and T2-weighted images, and with little or no edema.[38]

Treatment of MO is close observation. The lesion must mature and no longer show increased uptake on a bone scan before any surgical treatment, otherwise there will be extensive local recurrence. Maturation usually occurs within 6 months to 1 year.[36]

Compartment Syndrome

Compartment syndrome needs to be considered when thigh contusions occur. Compartment pressures should be measured if there is concern for elevated pressures. Most clinicians would take patients to the operating room if the compartment pressure was higher than 30 mm Hg.[14,39–41] That being said, Robinson and colleagues[42] recommend that athletes with muscle contusions with no femur fracture should be merely observed. All 6 of the cases in their series recovered well and returned to activity. Other reports of nonoperative management of elevated thigh compartment pressures have been reported.[43] Robinson and colleagues[42] proposed 3 reasons for this phenomenon of improvement despite elevated pressures: (1) the large volume of the quadriceps muscle; (2) its relatively elastic fascia; and (3) the direct proximal connection to the hip musculature, which allows extravasation of fluid out of the compartment. No study to date has randomized patients to surgery versus nonoperative care for elevated compartment pressures.

Mithofer and colleagues[44] note that although an absolute pressure threshold remains to be established for the thigh, their study demonstrated that pressures of greater than 70 mm Hg call for expedited surgical decompression to avoid complications. Moreover, such injuries without femur fracture are different from those with femur fractures. The study by Mithofer and colleagues[44] indicates that a differential pressure of less than 30 mm Hg may be a more useful clinical parameter than absolute compartment pressure. Patients with pressure less than 30 mm Hg, with lower injury severity scores, and without femur fracture did better when they developed anterior compartment syndrome of the thigh. Arterial injury needs to be considered if the patient is hypotensive or if bleeding continues after fasciotomy.[45] If surgical treatment is not performed, close observation is needed to prevent development of serious problems.

SUMMARY

Thigh contusions are a common injury in sports that can cause prolonged disability if not treated correctly. The knee needs to be placed in 120° of flexion for 24 hours, with limited NSAID use for the first 48 to 72 hours. Complications such as MO and compartment syndrome need to be considered.

REFERENCES

1. Fernandez WG, Yard EE, Comstock RD. Epidemiology of lower extremity injuries among U.S. high school athletes. Acad Emerg Med 2007;14(7):641–5.
2. Rechel JA, Yard EE, Comstock RD. An epidemiologic comparison of high school sports injuries sustained in practice and competition. J Athl Train 2008;43(2):197–204.
3. Ekstrand J, Hagglund M, Walden M. Epidemiology of muscle injuries in professional football (soccer). Am J Sports Med 2011;39(6):1226–32.
4. Jackson DW, Feagin JA. Quadriceps contusions in young athletes. Relation of severity of injury to treatment and prognosis. J Bone Joint Surg Am 1973;55(1):95–105.

5. Beyer R, Ingerslev J, Sorensen B. Muscle bleeds in professional athletes—diagnosis, classification, treatment and potential impact in patients with haemophilia. Haemophilia 2010;16(6):858–65.
6. Jarvinen TA, Jarvinen TL, Kaariainen M, et al. Muscle injuries: optimising recovery. Best Pract Res Clin Rheumatol 2007;21(2):317–31.
7. Charge SB, Rudnicki MA. Cellular and molecular regulation of muscle regeneration. Physiol Rev 2004;84(1):209–38.
8. Huard J, Li Y, Fu FH. Muscle injuries and repair: current trends in research. J Bone Joint Surg Am 2002;84(5):822–32.
9. Li Y, Huard J. Differentiation of muscle-derived cells into myofibroblasts in injured skeletal muscle. Am J Pathol 2002;161(3):895–907.
10. Toumi H, F'Guyer S, Best TM. The role of neutrophils in injury and repair following muscle stretch. J Anat 2006;208(4):459–70.
11. Foster W, Li Y, Usas A, et al. Gamma interferon as an antifibrosis agent in skeletal muscle. J Orthop Res 2003;21(5):798–804.
12. Ghaly A, Marsh DR. Ischaemia-reperfusion modulates inflammation and fibrosis of skeletal muscle after contusion injury. Int J Exp Pathol 2010;91(3):244–55.
13. Alonso A, Hekeik P, Adams R. Predicting a recovery time from the initial assessment of a quadriceps contusion injury. Aust J Physiother 2000;46(3):167–77.
14. An HS, Simpson JM, Gale S, et al. Acute anterior compartment syndrome in the thigh: a case report and review of the literature. J Orthop Trauma 1987;1(2): 180–2.
15. Mithofer K, Lhowe DW, Vrahas MS, et al. Clinical spectrum of acute compartment syndrome of the thigh and its relation to associated injuries. Clin Orthop Relat Res 2004;(425):223–9.
16. Lee JC, Mitchell AW, Healy JC. Imaging of muscle injury in the elite athlete. Br J Radiol 2012;85(1016):1173–85.
17. Megliola A, Eutropi F, Scorzelli A, et al. Ultrasound and magnetic resonance imaging in sports-related muscle injuries. Radiol Med 2006;111(6):836–45.
18. Hayashi D, Hamilton B, Guermazi A, et al. Traumatic injuries of thigh and calf muscles in athletes: role and clinical relevance of MR imaging and ultrasound. Insights Imaging 2012;3:591–601.
19. Fornage BD. Soft tissue masses: the underutilization of sonography. Semin Musculoskelet Radiol 1999;3(2):115–34.
20. Blankenbaker DG, Tuite MJ. Temporal changes of muscle injury. Semin Musculoskelet Radiol 2010;14(2):176–93.
21. Aronen JG, Garrick JG, Chronister RD, et al. Quadriceps contusions: clinical results of immediate immobilization in 120 degrees of knee flexion. Clin J Sport Med 2006;16(5):383–7.
22. Thorsson O, Lilja B, Nilsson P, et al. Immediate external compression in the management of an acute muscle injury. Scand J Med Sci Sports 1997;7(3): 182–90.
23. Ryan JB, Wheeler JH, Hopkinson WJ, et al. Quadriceps contusions. West Point update. Am J Sports Med 1991;19(3):299–304.
24. Smith C, Kruger MJ, Smith RM, et al. The inflammatory response to skeletal muscle injury: illuminating complexities. Sports Med 2008;38(11):947–69.
25. Prisk V, Huard J. Muscle injuries and repair: the role of prostaglandins and inflammation. Histol Histopathol 2003;18(4):1243–56.
26. Rahusen FT, Weinhold PS, Almekinders LC. Nonsteroidal anti-inflammatory drugs and acetaminophen in the treatment of an acute muscle injury. Am J Sports Med 2004;32(8):1856–9.

27. Hubbard TJ, Denegar CR. Does cryotherapy improve outcomes with soft tissue injury? J Athl Train 2004;39(3):278–9.

28. Puntel GO, Carvalho NR, Amaral GP, et al. Therapeutic cold: an effective kind to modulate the oxidative damage resulting of a skeletal muscle contusion. Free Radic Res 2011;45(2):125–38.

29. Schaser KD, Disch AC, Stover JF, et al. Prolonged superficial local cryotherapy attenuates microcirculatory impairment, regional inflammation, and muscle necrosis after closed soft tissue injury in rats. Am J Sports Med 2007;35(1):93–102.

30. Hurme T, Rantanen J, Kalimo H. Effects of early cryotherapy in experimental skeletal muscle injury. Oxford, UK: Blackwell; 1993.

31. Jarvinen M, Lehto M, Sorvari T, et al. Effect of some anti-inflammatory agents on the healing of ruptured muscle. A study in rats. Milano (Italy): Kurtis; 1992.

32. Levine WN, Bergfeld JA, Tessendorf W, et al. Intramuscular corticosteroid injection for hamstring injuries. A 13-year experience in the National Football League. Am J Sports Med 2000;28(3):297–300.

33. McGeary RP, Bennett AJ, Tran QB, et al. Suramin: clinical uses and structure-activity relationships. Mini Rev Med Chem 2008;8(13):1384–94.

34. Lustberg MB, Pant S, Ruppert AS, et al. Phase I/II trial of non-cytotoxic suramin in combination with weekly paclitaxel in metastatic breast cancer treated with prior taxanes. Cancer Chemother Pharmacol 2012;70(1):49–56.

35. Nozaki M, Li Y, Zhu J, et al. Improved muscle healing after contusion injury by the inhibitory effect of suramin on myostatin, a negative regulator of muscle growth. Am J Sports Med 2008;36(12):2354–62.

36. Sokunbi G, Fowler JR, Ilyas AM, et al. A case report of myositis ossificans traumatica in the adductor magnus. Clin J Sport Med 2010;20(6):495–6.

37. Koh ES, McNally EG. Ultrasound of skeletal muscle injury. Semin Musculoskelet Radiol 2007;11(2):162–73.

38. Armfield DR, Kim DH, Towers JD, et al. Sports-related muscle injury in the lower extremity. Clin Sports Med 2006;25(4):803–42.

39. Gorman PW, McAndrew MP. Acute anterior compartmental syndrome of the thigh following contusion. A case report and review of the literature. J Orthop Trauma 1987;1(1):68–70.

40. Rooser B, Bengtson S, Hagglund G. Acute compartment syndrome from anterior thigh muscle contusion: a report of eight cases. J Orthop Trauma 1991;5(1):57–9.

41. Colosimo AJ, Ireland ML. Thigh compartment syndrome in a football athlete: a case report and review of the literature. Med Sci Sports Exerc 1992;24(9): 958–63.

42. Robinson D, On E, Halperin N. Anterior compartment syndrome of the thigh in athletes—indications for conservative treatment. J Trauma 1992;32(2):183–6.

43. Riede U, Schmid MR, Romero J. Conservative treatment of an acute compartment syndrome of the thigh. Arch Orthop Trauma Surg 2007;127(4):269–75.

44. Mithoefer K, Lhowe DW, Vrahas MS, et al. Functional outcome after acute compartment syndrome of the thigh. J Bone Joint Surg Am 2006;88(4):729–37.

45. Suzuki T, Moirmura N, Kawai K, et al. Arterial injury associated with acute compartment syndrome of the thigh following blunt trauma. Injury 2005;36(1): 151–9.

Hip Pointers

Matthew Hall, DO[a],*, Jeffrey Anderson, MD, FACSM[b]

KEYWORDS

- Hip pointers • Iliac crest contusion • Hip injuries

KEY POINTS

- Hip pointers are contusions to the iliac crest and surrounding soft tissue.
- They are common injuries in contact sports, such as football, hockey, and rugby, particularly at the elite levels.
- Hip pointers can result in significant pain and decreased function affecting athletic performance and result in missed training and game participation.
- When the injury is recognized and diagnosed early, rapid treatment can allow for immediate return to sport as well as with a more rapid return to preinjury status.

INTRODUCTION

Hip pointers are contusions to the iliac crest and surrounding soft tissue.[1,2] They are common injuries in contact sports, such as football, hockey, and rugby, particularly at the elite levels.[1] Despite this, hip and pelvic rim injuries in young athletes have received considerably less attention than injuries to the knee, shoulder, and ankle.[1] Hip pointers can result in significant pain and decreased function affecting athletic performance and result in missed training and game participation. When the injury is recognized and diagnosed early, rapid treatment can allow for immediate return to sport as well as a more rapid return to preinjury status.

Hip pointers, also known in the literature as iliac crest contusions, were first described in the literature in 1966. At that time, it was proposed that hip pointer be used solely to describe a contusion to the iliac crest after direct blow to the area.[3] The pathology leading to pain can be subperiosteal edema or bleeding from nutrient vessels of the underlying bone or hematoma formation within the surrounding muscle. A healthy athletic population is also more susceptible due to the minimal amount of soft tissue between the iliac crest and the surface.[4] Another proposed anatomic explanation for this injury described in the literature is a compression of the abductor muscles against the ilium or iliac crest.[5]

[a] Primary Care Sports Medicine Fellow, Department of Family Medicine, University of Connecticut, 99 Woodland Street, Hartford, CT 06088, USA; [b] Division of Athletics, University of Connecticut, 505 Stadium Road, Unit 3204, Storrs, CT 06269, USA
* Corresponding author.
E-mail address: Mahall@stfranciscare.org

Clin Sports Med 32 (2013) 325–330
http://dx.doi.org/10.1016/j.csm.2012.12.010
0278-5919/13/$ – see front matter © 2013 Elsevier Inc. All rights reserved.

EPIDEMIOLOGY

Injuries to the hip and pelvic rim are less common compared with other injuries of the lower extremities, such as the knee and ankle.[1] The exact incidence rate of hip pointers has not been reported in the literature, and further epidemiologic studies are needed to determine the incidence and prevalence in an athletic population. There have been some studies looking at hip pointers and, more generally, hip and pelvic contusions within specific athletic populations.

Studies have shown that injuries to the hip region in high school athletes range from 5% to 9%,[6] and, therefore, the prevalence of hip pointers can be predicted to be significantly less because this number incorporates all injuries to the hip. An epidemiologic study of hip injuries in National Football League football players between the years 1997 and 2006 reported a total of 738 hip injuries with 33% reported as "contusions."[1] Hip contusions were the second most common injury behind general muscle strains. Of these hip contusions, 82 were reported as hip pointers, which accounted for 11% of the total hip injuries and 35% of total hip contusions during that time period.[1] The total incidence of hip pointers, when looking at all injuries to National Football League players between 1997 and 2006, was 0.3%. Although the treatment method was not reported in this study, the mean days lost from training was reported as 5.6 days.[1] This is a more significant amount of time missed from training than the authors have seen in their experience or heard about anecdotally.

A retrospective study of Australian football league draftees, spanning 7 years, reported "hip haematoma" as 4% of all injuries to the hip and groin.[7] It was among the top 10 most common injuries to the hip and groin in their population. The reported incidence in the Australian football cohort was slightly higher than American football, which could be speculated as due to the tackling aspect of the sport plus the lack of protective hip and iliac crest padding in that sport.

Ice hockey is another contact sport where hip pointers are more common. In a cohort of National Collegiate Athletic Association ice hockey players, hip/pelvis contusions have been reported as 2.4% of the total injuries during game play.[8] Again, the study did not separate out true hip pointers from the group of contusions at the hip and pelvis, making it difficult to state the exact rate of the injury in this particular population.

ANATOMY

There are many muscle origins and insertions at the iliac crest.[9] Posteriorly along the iliac crest, the gluteus medius originates. The quadratus lumborum originates from the 12th rib and inserts on the most medial aspect of the iliac crest. Also, on the medial portion of the iliac crest, a small portion of the latissimus dorsi inserts. On the anterior aspect of the crest, the iliacus muscle originates and runs inferiorly. The tensor fascia lata and sartorius muscles originate from the anterior superior iliac spine just below the most anterior portion of the iliac crest down to lateral and medial aspects of the knee, respectively. Portions of the external and internal oblique and transversus abdominis musculature come down to attach along the iliac crest as well. There are no major blood vessels between the iliac crest and the surface; any bleeding or hematoma formation comes from the muscles themselves or smaller branching vessels. Cutaneous branches of the iliohypogastric and ilioinguinal nerves innervate the superficial skin areas around the iliac crest itself. The lateral femoral cutaneous nerve does travel inferiorly on the ilium and becomes more superficial around the anterior superior iliac spine and could be affected by the injury mechanism itself or iatrogenically with injection treatment.

CLINICAL PRESENTATION

Athletes present after a direct blow to an unpadded area of the iliac crest, typically by an opposing player.[3] It is also possible to sustain the injury with a fall onto the hip during sport, reported in both soccer and skiing.[4] Hockey players often sustain the injury after a hard check into the boards.[5] Patients present with pain over the iliac crest associated with some difficulty ambulating.[10] If a true hematoma results, a fluctuant mass may be palpable.[10] These injuries can be extremely painful and debilitating.

CLINICAL EVALUATION

As with all injuries, a detailed history and physical examination are essential to proper diagnosis. Patients report significant pain over the lateral hip with decreased range of motion and decreased athletic performance. They may have an antalgic gait or an inability to bear weight, and they have tenderness to palpation over the iliac crest. Because the mechanism of injury for hip pointers is a direct blow, it differs from muscle strains or avulsion fractures of the hip, which typically result from rotational movements during participation[3] or an eccentric load that exceeds the strength of the myotendinous junction or tendon insertion.[6] Plain radiographs of the hip are generally not needed but can help rule out fractures or apophyseal avulsions in skeletally immature patients,[10] if clinical suspicion exists. This is an important consideration for high school and even collegiate athletes because the ischial tuberosity and anterior superior iliac spine can fuse as late as the 3rd decade of life.[6] In addition to musculoskeletal injuries, it is also crucial to rule intra-abdominal injuries, such as renal hematoma and splenic lacerations with a thorough abdominal examination.

CONSERVATIVE TREATMENT

To minimize bleeding and hematoma formation, initial attempts should concentrate on controlling bleeding and swelling.[5] Rapid direct compression with a wrap and ice are effective in reducing bleeding and swelling by causing vasoconstriction. If a significant hematoma is present, rarely an aspiration could be considered for pain relief and to prevent against heterotopic bone formation. One treatment protocol reported in the literature is to place athletes on crutches with severe hip pointers until the athlete is able to ambulate without a limp.[5] If oral analgesics are necessary, acetaminophen is preferable due to theoretic risk of increasing bleeding with nonsteroidal anti-inflammatory drugs or aspirin.[5] After pain improves and bleeding and/or swelling controlled, a rehabilitation program concentrating on hip abduction strengthening and hip range of motion.[5]

TREATMENT WITH LOCAL ANESTHETIC AND CORTICOSTEROID

Treatment of hip pointers should be dictated by individual athletes and their health care professionals, keeping in mind the particular athletic setting. Typically, pain relief and desire for return to play often drive decision making for elite athletes and their providers. The use of local anesthetic for return to play is common in select circumstances in sports, such as American football and Australian football, to allow for continued participation. It is generally believed safe, although there are few data regarding this practice.[11]

The author's preferred treatment for hip pointers, in a National Collegiate Athletic Association division I institution, is to inject the hip pointer immediately after diagnosis (**Figs. 1** and **2**). Once the diagnosis is made, the area of maximum tenderness is localized along the iliac crest. A combination of dexamethasone (of 2 mL) and 2% lidocaine

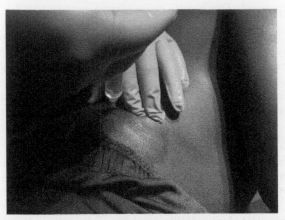

Fig. 1. At the point of maximum tenderness, the needle tip is guided down to the iliac crest the retracted slightly to inject around the periosteum.

or 0.5% bupivacaine (6 mL to 8 mL) is used. This method includes the use of corticosteroid to help with recovery. Although there are no controlled studies to support the use of corticosteroid, it is generally accepted within the sports medicine community. At the point of maximum tenderness, the needle tip is guided down to the iliac crest and then retracted slightly with the intent of injecting into the periosteum. Several milliliters are injected into the point of maximal tenderness and then the remainder is injected along the iliac crest anteriorly and posteriorly. Athletes generally feel relief quickly and are able to return to game participation almost immediately in the majority of cases. On return to play in this situation, the area is further protected with additional padding. One study, with a sample of 71 injections, reported that 75% of rugby players found iliac crest contusion injection to be very helpful, with the remaining 25% finding it somewhat helpful.[11]

COMPLICATIONS

Hip pointers can be extremely painful at the time of injury; however, if treated appropriately, there are minimal long-term concerns.[5] There have been reports of

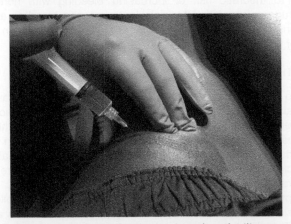

Fig. 2. Once the point of maximum tenderness is injected on the iliac crest, inject anteriorly then posteriorly along the iliac crest.

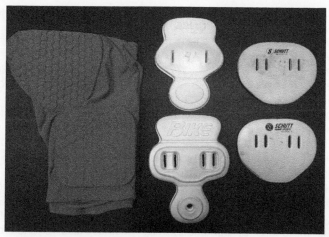

Fig. 3. Examples of hip padding used in the prevention of hip pointers.

developing bone exostosis or periostitis if not treated properly and in a timely manner.[10] Inadvertently, a sensory nerve block of the lateral femoral cutaneous nerve could be performed,[12] resulting in self-limiting sensation loss over the lateral thigh down to the knee. Other rare complications that have been reported in the literature are significant bleeding and bruising postgame down into the scrotum—this was a single occurrence in a sample of 71 hip pointer injections.[11] It is difficult to say if the bruising and bleeding were worsened by the injection itself or if the injury progressed because the player was able to participate despite the injury. Another more long-term complication, reported in the same study of rugby players, was a single report of chronic nonpainful lumps at the site of the injection.[11] Again, these were rare occurrences and it is difficult to state direct cause-and-effect relationship with the injection itself. Furthermore, reporting of complications from hip pointer injections is needed to determine complications and rates of complications. The majority of those who received the injection reported that they would opt to have the injection in the future if needed.[11] The benefits seem to outweigh the risks with hip pointer injections in a properly selected patient population with a definitive diagnosis. The injections are most useful for the population of high-level or elite athletes.

INJURY PREVENTION

Hip injuries in general can be decreased by increasing core stability and strength, in addition to properly fitting protective equipment.[13] There are multiple hip pads on the market aimed at helping to prevent against hip pointers. These include spandex shorts with padding built into the lateral hip as well as external pads that fit under an athlete's outer uniform garments (**Fig. 3**). In searching the literature, there does not seem to be any data supporting a decrease in hip injuries as a result of padding. Athletes who have sustained a hip pointer should have their equipment and padding inspected to ensure proper fitting to help prevent future injury.[5]

REFERENCES

1. Feeley BT, Powell JW, Muller MS, et al. Hip injuries and labral tears in the national football league. Am J Sports Med 2008;36(11):2187–95.

2. Waite BL, Krabak BJ. Examination and treatment of pediatric injuries of the hip and pelvis. Phys Med Rehabil Clin N Am 2008;19(2):305–18, ix.
3. Blazina ME. The "hip-pointer", a term to describe a specific kind of athletic injury. Calif Med 1967;106(6):450.
4. Martinez J. Hip Pointers. Medscape Reference. 2011 12/13/2011 9/2012.
5. LaPrade RF, Wijdicks CA, Griffith CJ. Division I intercollegiate ice hockey team coverage. Br J Sports Med 2009;43(13):1000–5.
6. Anderson K, Strickland SM, Warren R. Hip and groin injuries in athletes. Am J Sports Med 2001;29(4):521–33.
7. Gabbe BJ, Bailey M, Cook JL, et al. The association between hip and groin injuries in the elite junior football years and injuries sustained during elite senior competition. Br J Sports Med 2010;44(11):799–802.
8. Agel J, Dompier TP, Dick R, et al. Descriptive epidemiology of collegiate men's ice hockey injuries: National Collegiate Athletic Association Injury Surveillance System, 1988-1989 through 2003-2004. J Athl Train 2007;42(2):241–8.
9. Schuenke M, Shulte E, Schumacher U. Thieme: Atlas of anatomy: general anatomy and musculoskeletal system. New York: Thieme; 2006.
10. DeLee J, Drez D, Miller M. DeLee and Drez's Orthopaedic sports medicine. 3rd edition. Philadelphia, PA: Saunders; 2010. p. 1458–9.
11. Orchard JW, Steet E, Massey A, et al. Long-term safety of using local anesthetic injections in professional rugby league. Am J Sports Med 2010;38(11):2259–66.
12. Orchard JW. Benefits and risks of using local anaesthetic for pain relief to allow early return to play in professional football. Br J Sports Med 2002;36(3):209–13.
13. Kovacevic D, Mariscalco M, Goodwin RC. Injuries about the hip in the adolescent athlete. Sports Med Arthrosc 2011;19(1):64–74.

Index

Note: Page numbers of article titles are in **boldface** type.

Clin Sports Med 32 (2013) 331–337
http://dx.doi.org/10.1016/S0278-5919(13)00011-2
0278-5919/13/$ – see front matter © 2013 Elsevier Inc. All rights reserved.

sportsmed.theclinics.com

Moving?

Make sure your subscription moves with you!

To notify us of your new address, find your **Clinics Account Number** (located on your mailing label above your name), and contact customer service at:

Email: journalscustomerservice-usa@elsevier.com

800-654-2452 (subscribers in the U.S. & Canada)
314-447-8871 (subscribers outside of the U.S. & Canada)

Fax number: 314-447-8029

Elsevier Health Sciences Division
Subscription Customer Service
3251 Riverport Lane
Maryland Heights, MO 63043

*To ensure uninterrupted delivery of your subscription, please notify us at least 4 weeks in advance of move.

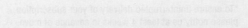

Printed and bound by CPI Group (UK) Ltd, Croydon, CR0 4YY

03/10/2024

01040442-0012